Carl & Shelia Millender

THE

RAINBOW DIET

Your Journey to Great Health

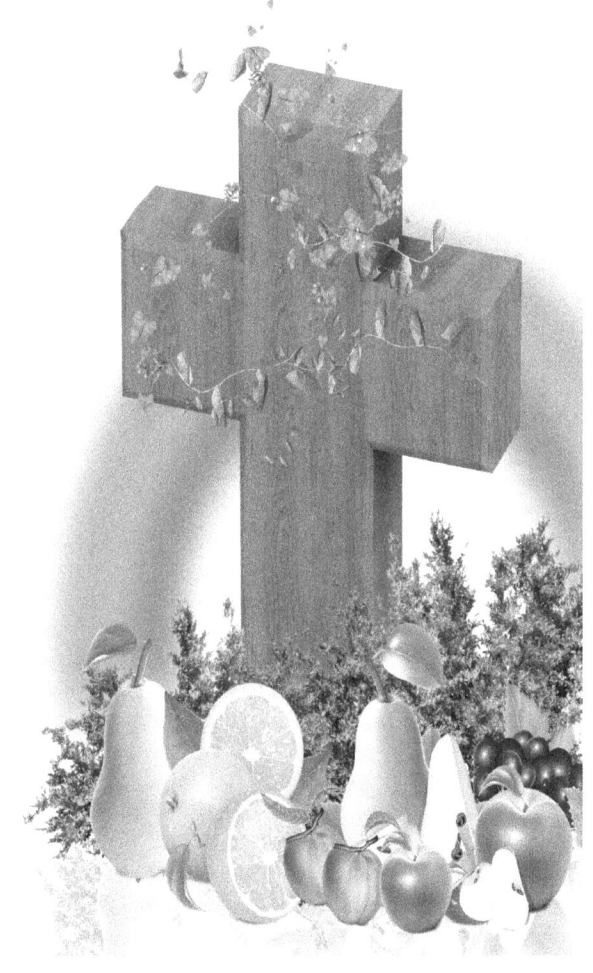

The Rainbow Diet

Your Journey to great health

By Carl and Shelia Millender

Published by M&M Herbs, Inc.

M&M Herbs Inc. Products are available at special discounts for bulk purchase, for sales promotions, fundraising, and educational needs.

For details write M&M Herbs Inc.3737 Holcomb Bridge Road Norcross, GA 30092, or call (678) 698-1970.

The Rainbow Diet by Carl and Shelia Millender

Published by M&M Herbs Inc.3737 Holcomb Bridge Rd. Norcross, GA 30092
www.therainbowdiet.org

Unless otherwise noted, all Scripture quotations are from the New King James or NIV versions of the Bible.

Cover design by Mariacristina Romano.

Copyright © 2006, 2007

First Edition, 2006

Revised Edition 2007

Third Edition 2014

Dedication

My deepest appreciation........... to Dr. Sebe of the Fig Tree in the Dominican Republic and Dr. William Richardson of the Atlanta Preventive Medicine Clinic, in Georgia. It is through your journeys that our journey began.

Also we love you, Mom. You are our favorite author. It was only when you finished your first book that we knew it was a possible task.

To our Dads: Without your hard work none of the opportunities (education, travels, and lifestyle) in our life would have come as easy.

Table of Contents

Preface

It is my sincere hope that everyone in the world will have perfect health, but the truth is that will never happen. Many of us are born with severe problems from birth. However, many of us are born happy healthy babies. It is only after years of torturing our bodies with horrible foods that our bodies begin to fail us. This book is for those of us who just never knew what to do with this terrific instrument called the human body. This instrument produces miracles every day. It can turn an apple into blood, a mushroom into bone and oxygen into life. In fact, the human body produces miracles all day long and most of us never stop to thank God for these wonderful occurrences.

I once met an atheist. He believed in something similar to the big bang theory and he thought that everyone just simply evolved out of nothing. I asked him, "What was more complex, the human body or the space shuttle?" He kind of just looked at me. I nudged on. I said, "Which do you think is the hardest to make? Let me give you a clue." I told him. "We will never be able to create a human body out of nothing, but we created the space shuttle over 20 years ago." I asked him, "Do you believe whatever in a billion years that a series of events could simply happen and magically, a space shuttle would appear out of a cloud of dust." He never spoke to me again but I think he got the point.   The truth is that just about any levelheaded scientist will tell you that the human body is a magnificent creation not a mishap.

Our body is so complex that only a Great Being could have assembled it and only that Being could have made an instruction manual for it. That being was God himself and the manual is called the Bible. It teaches on three platforms: mind, body, and soul. This book "The Rainbow Diet," primarily addresses the "body" part and what God has said we should do to maintain it.

In the summer of 1988, I had my first experience as a foreign missionary spreading the word of Jesus Christ to the exterior of a country in South America called Paraguay. For the most part we ministered in a small town called Iguasu. 95% of the homes had no electricity, running water, or indoor bathrooms. Only one hotel and a few restaurants had anything that resembled modern civilization. Needless to say the food was greatly different. Most people did not have refrigerators so what they ate was made and served the same day. There were very few cows; in fact I only remember seeing two. Most people had goats. For weeks all I drank was fresh goat's milk and oven made bread. My clothes were washed in the river and I saw more "outhouse"- type holes in the ground than I care to remember. One reason was because I found myself going to the bathroom much more than normal. It seemed to have something to do with the foods they were serving me. My body started responding by having more bowel movements. At that time I remember thinking, "This is annoying," but the other side effect I experienced was awesome. My allergies, which I had possessed as long as I could remember, simply disappeared. So much that I didn't want to leave once the mission's trip ended. The only reason I came back to the States was because I had promised my parents I would complete college.

Lots of things happened that changed my life that summer. However, the primary thing that happened was I realized on a first hand basis that life was not the same in the United States in other areas of the world. I didn't have to watch TV to be entertained. There were no televisions in this small town of eight hundred or so residents. There was only one radio station and the only language they spoke was a country-style dialectic mixture of a Spanish and Iguaçu Indian tongue; so I couldn't understand what they were saying anyway. During this time I grew closer to God than I ever thought possible. All my life I had worried about why I wasn't as rich as other people I knew, and why they could do things and have things I couldn't. I remember saying to God what a fool I had been to not see I was already rich. I lived in the United States, the greatest country in the world. Our poorest person was rich compared to the people I was living with at that time. However, I failed to realize something very important, maybe the most important thing. What they lacked in possessions and money they made up for in diet. I don't think I ever felt better physically in my life.

It wasn't until many years later that I realized the physical feeling I had encountered in Paraguay was not by chance. What I had experienced was a closer encounter to the food and healthy lifestyle God had intended us to all have. It is something I am always in search of; hopefully, you will be, too.

Father, I pray every soul in the world can somehow benefit from this word you have given me to place in this book (as well as the word you gave Moses on the mountain and all of the great writers in the instruction manual we call the Bible.) though You know it as simply Your Word. We want to experience that true feeling of Godly health - the way you designed our bodies to feel. Open everyone's minds and pull back the veil of deception from the "Rainmen." - Carl Millender

Introduction

First of all, I'd like to thank you for allowing me to share with you this small part of your life and for taking this important step in your journey for good health. The things I will be presenting to you may seem shocking. It may even be unbelievable, but I promise I will support much of what you read with evidence.

Okay, let's get started. Some of my best friends are from New York. New Yorkers are truly some of the best people in the world. However, New York is one of my least favorite places to visit. During my first two visits, I witnessed a purse snatching where a bandit almost knocked me down making his getaway. Next, I saw a car being broken into right in front of me. The guy looked at me, as if to say "who is this person that has the audacity to look at me and you had better mind your own business." And thirdly, the tires of the van I was traveling in were stolen while it was parked in a "secured" garage. (I believe the security guard got them.) So you can understand why whenever I get a chance to poke a joke at New Yorkers, I do. So what the heck, there is no time like the present.

One glorious day in heaven Saint Peter was tending to his duties, guarding the Great Pearly Gates, when out of nowhere, "poof," a group of people appeared. All of them had similar accents and attitudes demanding Saint Peter to allow them to enter heaven. Now of course Saint Pete first graciously asked each one of them for their names and where they were from. They each gave their information and to Saint Peter's amazement they were all from New York City. Now Peter had allowed people from New York into the Gates before but never in so large a group. This would truly be rare. So Saint Peter tells everyone to "hold on" and he trots off in a saintly way to the great throne of God.

Once there, Peter tells God about the odd group of New Yorkers at the Pearly Gates and asks if he should let them in.

God looks through His big book and sees that He was expecting a church bus from New York later that day. "Oh they're early but let them in and tell them I have prepared a beautiful place for them."

So, Saint Peter trots back off in a saintly way. A short time later Peter comes running back to the throne this time in a not so saintly way. As he runs, he's yelling "Father, Father they're gone, they're gone!" As Peter stops at the throne (out of breath) he says one last time, "They're gone!"   God looks down at Peter and says "Who's gone Peter? The New Yorkers?"   Peter looks up at God and says, "No God, the Gates, the Pearly Gates are gone!"

I like to use that story not just because it's funny and cute but also because it symbolizes the state of our health. If you don't understand, let me explain. Hopefully, when you're done reading this book, you will not only understand but "over stand. "There are groups of people knocking at the Pearly Gates of our bodies (our teeth). Just like the New Yorkers at the Gates in the story, who Saint Peter thought looked "a little suspect," these people look a little suspicious in one way or another. They are waiting to rob you of your health. Likewise, if we turn our attention for a moment, something disastrous can happen. I like to call these unruly people "Rainmen.

The Rainstorm

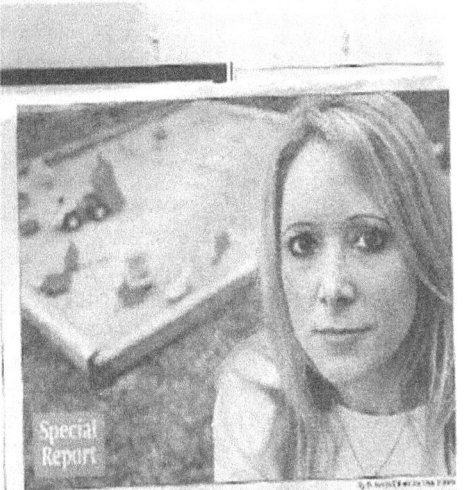

Seeing Roche: Debbie Banner blames [Accutane for her son's] severe birth defects. She took the acne drug in 1995 and found herself "constantly thinking about dying." Her son, now 8, has cerebral palsy.

Drugmaker rebuffed call to monitor users

Lawsuits say Accutane caused birth defects, depression and deaths

By Revin McCoy
USA TODAY

The maker of Accutane, a controversial acne medication, disregarded a company doctor's recommendation that users of the drug be monitored for signs of depression and that a warning to that effect be added to the drug's U.S. label, allegations in a federal court case show.

The Florida lawsuit against the company, Hoffmann-La Roche, charges that the Swiss drug giant ignored the warning after its marketing officials argued that such an alert could scare doctors away from prescribing the drug. The doctor's recommendation and the marketing debate sketched in legal files have not been previously publicized.

There has been no official finding that links Accutane to depression or other psychiatric illnesses. Roche says the drug is effective when used properly. Nonetheless, a senior Roche official, testifying in a pretrial deposition for the Florida case, said the firm's internal analysis showed Accutane "probably caused" depression and other psychiatric illnesses in some patients, according to a summary of the deposition in a court brief.

The mental debate alleged in the case comes to light after a U.S. Food and Drug

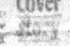

Please see COVER STORY next page

Have you ever been riding down the street in a rainstorm and you see you are about to drive through a rain puddle just as your car skids and loses control? For the most part, these puddles are harmless but for some, they prove to be deadly. Each year thousands of people drive through what they thought were small puddles of water and the next thing they know, their cars stall or worse they and their cars are being carried in another direction by the rainwater. For many, their car turns into a watery grave.

In today's society, there are groups of people tell us it is okay to eat certain foods or it is okay to take certain drugs. Some of the things they tell us it's okay to do are things we have serious doubts about. These guys -"THE RAINMEN" are also known as doctor, pharmacist, grocery store, FDA, and sometimes even pastor. Every time we take a pill that we haven't had before, just before we place it in our mouths, we may say to ourselves, "I hope this doesn't hurt me. I hope I don't die because I swallowed this." Eventually we say to ourselves, "Well, my doctor says it's okay," and we flip it into our mouths anyway. We've all done it at some time or another and fortunately we're all still here, but the story doesn't always end so delightful.

Debbie Banner wishes she had listened to that little voice in her head in 1995. In the December 7, 2004 issue of USA Today, she along with a large group of other people blamed Accutane for their constant depression and for birth defects like her son's cerebral palsy.

A USA Today article dated February 1, 2005 states two out of every hundred children taking antidepressants ended up thinking of ways to commit suicide. That's interesting. Imagine giving your child.... something to keep him from being depressed and instead he gets even more depressed and now wants to commit suicide. The article goes on to say that these reactions are not caused by just one particular antidepressant but all of them have been the subjects of stories reporting similar affects.

Parents all over the world were wondering why their precious child slit his wrist wide open while he was on drugs which were supposed to stop his depression.

In 1989 I had a similar experience with drugs. I came down with some sort of a cold and my doctor gave me an antibiotic. The prescribed dosage was two tablets every 6 hours. As I was about to put the tablets in my mouth something told me, "Don't do it."

Have you ever felt like if I do this I might be in trouble but if I don't, I may also be in trouble -you know, stuck in a situation you don't want to be in? I was so sick, I chose to straddle the fence. I compromised with my conscience and took only one tablet. About 6 hours later I was supposed to take another dose, but I couldn't because within an hour after I had taken the first pill my throat was nearly completely swollen shut. The only way I could breathe was to lay flat on my back with my head hanging off the side of the bed. This allowed a small amount of air to move through my throat and into my lungs. I wanted to go to the doctor but I couldn't go anywhere; every time I tried to lift my head I felt like I was suffocating.

Isn't it funny how we go to doctors and when they mess up, we go right back for them to "practice medicine" on us all over again?

It was winter break at college. Because I was sick and had to work, I did not make the five hour drive home. None of my classmates had stayed behind. They had all gone home for the break. Even if someone had been close by, I couldn't have called him or her on the phone because I couldn't talk. They wouldn't have known to whom they were speaking; of course, that was before the time of caller ID. So I sat there for two whole days praying that I wouldn't die. Gradually my throat opened back up and I made a promise to myself never to take any medicine again unless I had studied it and knew more about it. I was one of the lucky ones, but there are far too many who aren't.

On July 26, 2000, the most noted medical journal in the United States - JAMA- the Journal of America Medical Association ran an article by Dr.Starfield of Johns Hopkins University. The article revealed startling information. Every year more than 250,000 people in the U.S. are killed by their physician who was "practicing medicine on them."

Worldwide, that's easily more than 300,000. Don't get me wrong there are some very good doctors out there but these numbers are astounding. More than 300,000 people die per year. Some of you didn't even blink at that number. Let me put this into perspective for you.

but the data was hard to reference as it was not in peer-reviewed journal. Now it is published in JAMA which is the most widely circulated medical periodical in the world.

DEATHS PER YEAR:
1. 12,000 ·····unnecessary surgery 8
2. 7,000 ·····medication errors in hospitals 9
3. 20,000 ····other errors in hospitals 10
4. 80,000 ····infections in hospitals 10
5. 106,000 ···non-error, negative effects of drugs 2

250,000 deaths per year from iatrogenic...death induced

On September 11, 2001, roughly 2,800 people were killed by terrorists in the U.S.

In the Gulf War and Iraq together to date just over 10,000 of our troops have been

killed in the line of duty. During the entire Vietnam War 56,000 of our troops were

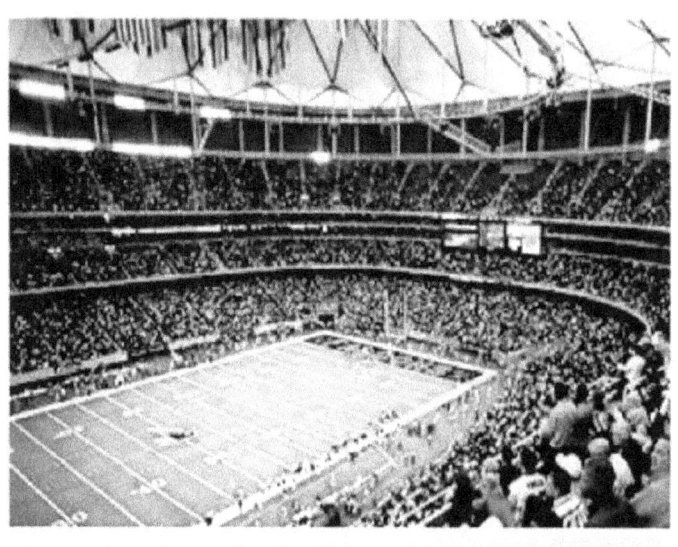

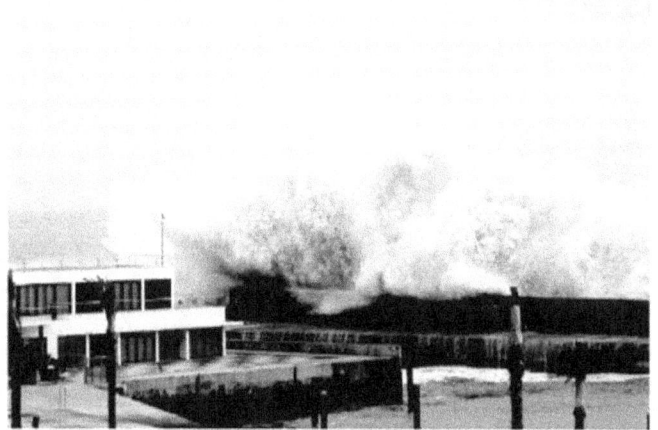

killed. If you were to add up every plane crash that has ever happened in the United states since Vietnam you still wouldn't come anywhere near 300,000. Let's throw in a "sold out" Georgia Dome which seats 71,250 and a "sold out" Turner Field which seats 50,091. Now you're getting close to the number.

In fact the only single occurrence in recent history that gets close to this number was the December 2004 tsunami, where 290,000 people lost their lives. For the tsunami, we had "tsunami relief." People from all over the world sent help. There was news coverage for months and still to this very moment we are helping people there reestablish their lives and homes.

During Vietnam, we had protests and flag burnings. After 9/11, we took over a country and bombed another to smithereens. The government halted flights all over the world and grounded every flight over the United States and Canada something that had never been attempted before. 1500 flights over Canada, 4200 over the US and 239 flights over the ocean on their way to North America. We've got memorial after memorial all across our nation for almost every soldier who has died in one on these wars, yet I bet you still didn't blink an eye or raise your hands in amazement when you read doctors kill over 300,000 per year.

Most of you still don't understand. It's not just 300,000 people. - It's 300,000 people every year!!!!!!!! That's 300,000 in —1989, 1990, 1991, 1992, 1993, 1994, 1995, 1996, 1997, 1998, 1999, 2000, 2001, 2002, 2003, 2004, 2005, and 2006. How much longer are we going to let this go on???

Let me go a little further, let us see who else is knocking at our "Pearly Gates."

It's not only doctors and pharmacists doing the knocking. It's all around us. How about the last time you were in the grocery store? Did you hear anyone knocking while you were there? No? Well you should have. You know when you were standing there over the grapes trying to decide which bag to grab. "Should I get the one that says seeded and organic which came from across town or should I get the one that says seedless which cost 20 cents less and somehow came all the way from Chile?"   So you take a sample bite and go "Hum, no crunchy feeling, I choose this one." Or worse, has your local grocery store simply stopped carrying the seeded grapes because no one buys them any-more?

Hasn't that light ever gone off in your mind that said, "Now how did someone take all those seeds out of those grapes? I mean.....God didn't make them that way so someone had to take them out? I mean... How do they reproduce themselves? "Come on, I know you've asked yourself that question. The most important part of the grape is missing and we don't even ask the grocery manager where he put all of the grape's seeds.

In the health food store, a bottle of grape seed extract costs around $30. We pay it because it contains some of the strongest antioxidants known to man. It deters cancer. It gets rid of free radical damage that destroys your eyesight and its anti-aging properties are amazing. If we just bought the organic seeded grapes for 50 cents more we could avoid a great deal of pain, save a great deal of money and be much healthier.

Everyone reading this has bought or attempted to buy health food at one time or another. Haven't we all been shocked by how much health food costs? On average, the health food costs about 20% more but we never stop to think about how much money it can save us in the long run.

Healthy cost 20% more

Organic vs. Other

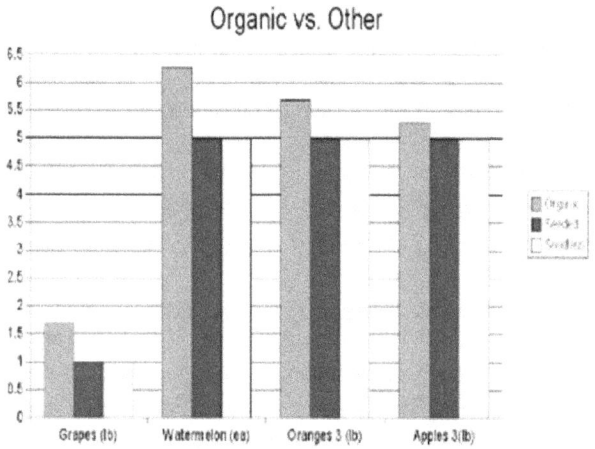

The "Rainmen" tell us its okay to eat biogenetically modified products and we eat them without even questioning it. We never stop to ask why some company would spend millions of dollars to create a grape without seeds. Well, I did a little research. Guess what I found out? It's all Big Business "$$$." They're not thinking about your health. They're thinking about their pockets; otherwise they would have left the seeds inside the grapes. The biogenetic companies figured out they could sell seeds that would deter insects, wildlife and plant diseases. This is all great but oh by the way, the grapes don't produce new seeds. Hatsa nifty trick. So....farmers wanting to grow new grapevines would have to come back each year to buy more seeds over and over again. Yeah, that's right more money! They weren't thinking about your health or your eating enjoyment; they weren't even thinking about your environment. For decades, scientists have argued over the effects of cross breeding plants. Some say there is no major impact on the environment and others disagree.

advancement is in the Sept. 17 issue of Science.

Genes from biotech grass scatter for miles

Genetically engineered grass developed for use on golf courses can spread its modified genes for miles, carried by ultra-light pollen particles, report a team of Environmental Protection Agency researchers. And another government agency, the U.S. Department of Agriculture, says it already has plans to conduct an environmental impact investigation into the potential effects of the plant, which will keep it off the market for a year or more. Creeping bentgrass, created by Scotts Co. and modified to resist weed killers, pollinated grasses as far as 13 miles away, says a report in this week's *Proceedings of the National Academy of Sciences.* The findings appear to support arguments that it will be difficult to control genetically modified plants from interbreeding with surrounding plants to create new and unanticipated hybrids.

An article in USA Today featured a story about bent grass created for golf courses to resist weed killers. This grass had pollinated grasses as far as 13 miles away. The EPA feared that it would be difficult to control this grass from interbreeding with surrounding plants because it could create new unanticipated hybrids. You see, plants don't just mate in a certain area. They mate with plants in all the areas around them as far as the wind, birds or bees will carry their pollen. Now, not only does this affect plants, it affects the surrounding ecosystem. Hold that thought! I'll come back to it.

Every day we all encounter things like this. Sometimes we question them but never for long. This thought pattern is a deadly symptom of an even more deadly disease. As a consultant who specializes in business and health, I see it every day. It's called "collective reasoning" or in layman's terms "They are all doing it so it must be okay." It's the exact opposite of what we tell our children everyday.

"Little Johnny, why did you roll the neighbor's trees with toilet paper?"

"Dad, all the kids were doing it. It's Halloween. It'll come out eventually."

" Johnny that's stupid. If your friends jump off a bridge, are you going to jump off it, too?"

Does that sound familiar? We think just because everyone else is eating seedless grapes, we should eat them, too.

In a big corporation it sounds more like this: "Mr. Manager, your company loses $400,000 every year in lost labor because you let your employees leave 5 minutes early every day. Why do you continue to do that?" Well sir, all the other departments were doing it and it's been going on so long.....So I figured why go against the grain?"

People wake up. It's to the point now that when I walk into a company or a sick person's room, one of the first things I ask them is: "Are you ready to make a change?" Almost always the response is an apprehensive "yes." Then in each of their own unique way, they ask me, "What kind of a change?" Then I look them in the eyes and say, "Whatever it takes?" Whatever it takes to save your company or your body. Every time I repeat this phrase, I get a pause. Sometimes it's short, and sometimes it's long. It's as if they believe it's okay to keep doing the same thing over and over even if it's killing them; even if it's costing their company $400,000 a year.   What are the effects? For the company I just mentioned, the shareholder's stocks were decreasing in value. The product prices were going up, causing the doctors who use those products to pay more money. The excess spending ultimately raises the cost of our health care.

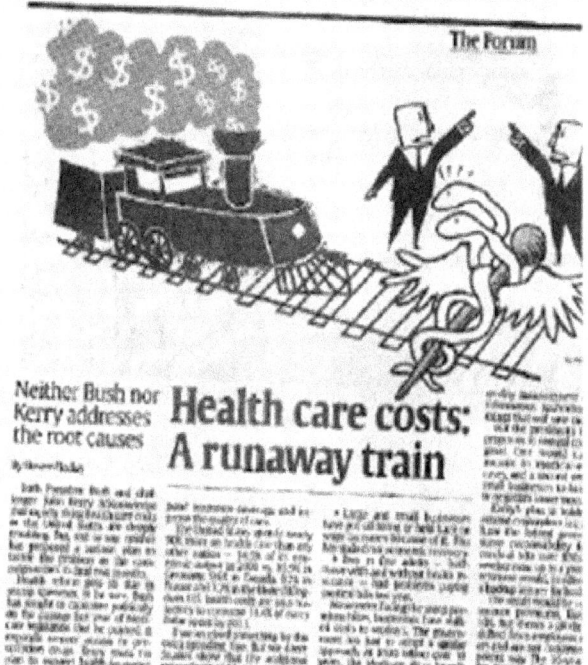

For your body the stakes are much higher; high blood pressure, diabetes, and heart disease are household words when they should rarely be heard of. How much more are you willing to pay? Are you willing to pay with your life? That's a big statement but are you going to keep living your life the same way because everyone else is doing it? Are you ready to do whatever it takes to save yourself or do you want to keep drowning in this flood of bad health we have in America? Are you willing to do whatever it takes to save yourself from the "Rainmen?" If your answer is "yes, I want to be saved," then repeat these words out loud. "Whatever It Takes!" I don't care where you are, even if you are in church or the library. Come on, one more time. "Whatever It Takes!"

God's Rainbow Diet

Okay, let's get started..... The Bible says that; during the time of the great flood, it rained for forty days and forty nights. That was enough to flood the earth to the point that ocean fossils are still being found at some of the highest mountain ranges in the United States. It doesn't take long for flood waters to rise, but just in case you don't know or can't feel it, it's been raining on your health for more than 40 days and 40 nights. But just like God gave Noah the Ark to save himself and family, He has provided a lifesaver for you, too. Let's call this lifesaver the "Rainbow Diet."

I don't profess to be a preacher, even though I feel God has placed a strong calling on my life to help others. At times, I might sound like I'm preaching but it's just because everything about taking care of our bodies is found in the Bible. The Bible is like an instruction manual for our mind, body and soul. Whether you believe it or not, they are all connected.

I've chosen "The Rainbow Diet" as the title of this not so new habit in eating because it symbolizes a great deal of things which I feel are important in this battle for good health. The colors represent all of the different people who desire to be healthy.

The Rainbow has been adopted by the gay and lesbian communities as their international symbol. They are a group of people who greatly need to hear this information. A large amount of them claim not to have any natural attraction to the opposite sex. Something I feel has a great deal to do with hormonal imbalance. Many make statements like, "I feel like the opposite sex inside." So, they are attracted to the same sex or simply are not attracted to the opposite sex. This may have a lot to do with excessive hormones placed in foods and pharmaceutical products and high levels of BPA (bisphenol A) found in plastics many of us use.

In regards to rainbows, I've always heard that there was a pot of gold at the end of each one. At the end of this book, hopefully you'll find your pot of golden health.

Most importantly the rainbow represents the most popular of all of God's Promises. After the great flood, God promised Noah and you (his descendants) to never flood the entire earth with water again. He placed a rainbow in the sky so that after every storm, just in case you were getting worried, we would remember that it would never again be as bad as it was in the days of Noah.

There is joy after the storm or as my good friend, the great motivational speaker, Keith L.Brown says, "Every setback is a setup for a come-back." I like that image and I hope, after reading this book, your state of health will never again be as bad as it is today.

Some of you just said to yourselves, "I'm in pretty good health. What's he talking about?" Well, let's just take a look at that.

Are the "Rainmen" ruining your health? Canyon feel it? Just put your hands on your head. Is there water up there? Is your hair drenched? Some of you are probably wondering why I ask, "is your hair wet?" Before you answer those questions, let me explain....

I'm a big movie buff. In fact, in my spare time, I like to both professionally produce movies as well as watch them. One of my favorite all-time movie lines was said by a small child near the end of the famous movie starring Oprah Winfrey and Danny Glover called, "The Color Purple." In the middle of this very serious scene as Harpo is repairing the ceiling of the Juke Joint, there's a thunderstorm moving closer. A small child sees the hole in the ceiling and makes the statement: "It's gone rain on yon head. "Do you remember that line? The entire group of people where I saw it broke out into wild laughter. But the truth was if the hole didn't get fixed rain would be falling on their heads. So what if I were to tell you, "It's been raining on your head since you were born." But because of collective reasoning, you have not seen it and you don't know that you're close to drowning; and many of your family members have already gone under.

You still don't feel the water from the "Rainmen" all around you? Well... let me help you: you get frequent headaches? Are you experiencing memory loss? Are you balding? Do you have premature gray hair? Is your vision weak or weakening? Do you have acne? How about sinus issues? Do you go around hacking or making weird noises with your throat? Or do you have a slight cough that you have had for years adjust can't seem to get rid of? How about bad breath? Is everyone offering you a piece of gum or a mint everywhere you go? What about tooth decay? Gum disease? Did you know animals in the wild don't have either and they never brush their teeth! Do you bleed every time you brush your teeth? Is your tongue milky white instead of pink? Does it look like the Rocky Mountains when it should be smooth? Do you ever have fever blisters? How's your hearing? Your sense of smell? Your sense of taste are you losing it? Are your eyes discolored? Did you know there are only two true eye colors - brown and blue? If you answered yes to any of those questions, you better pull out an umbrella because, "It's raining on your head."

Now, let's see if you need a towel to dry off or do you really need a lifesaver vest (this book) to keep from drowning. Do you have skin rashes, psoriasis, eczema, moles, liver spots, dry skin, or vitiligo? If you are a person of color, is your skin starting to look like Michael Jackson's? Are you plagued with persistent heavy coughs, obesity, anorexia, back problems, carpal tunnel, fatigue, or depression?   Get a bucket.

Or is it much worse? Do you have high blood pressure, diabetes, heart disease or cancer? Call out the Marines. Hurry up! Get out of the Ocean that's forming around you! Your lungs are filling with water! Death is not far away! Some of you have just a few breaths left and don't even know it. The rest of you know it but can't see which way God threw the life preserver. Well, today I hope you'll find it. So listen up.

Let's address how you got in this situation first, because if you don't understand that, then you'll never understand how to get out of it. One of the most popular stories in the Old Testament is the story of creation, starring God, the almighty; Adam, God's first version of man; Eve, the improved version; and the deceiving serpent, better known as Satan. The story begins after God has placed Adamant Eve in this beautiful garden called Eden (Genesis 2:16, 17) God tells Adam & Eve that they can have anything they want in the garden but do not eat of the forbidden tree of knowledge of good and evil.

17 "But you must not eat from the tree of the knowledge of good and evil, for when you eat obit you will surely die."

We all know this story and how it ends but just think about this part for a moment. I don't think any of us ever read much into this part. How did we come to call this tree "the tree of knowledge of good and evil" and why is that name significant? "Knowledge" sounds like a good thing to have but under these circumstances it clearly wasn't. The serpent even uses the thought of knowledge being good thing to lure Eve into taking a bite of food that she knows she shouldn't. (Genesis 3:5)

5 "For God knows that when you eat of it your eyes will be opened, and you will be like God, knowing good and evil."

I don't think for a minute that God just said "I've got to give them a random test to see if they will obey or not." I believe there was nothing ran-doom about it at all. He didn't say, "Hum should tell them never to cross this line." "How about never say my name backwards." No, he said, "Do not eat of the tree of knowledge of good and evil."

God who created over a million complex species of living organisms has a perfect order for things? God knew there was one tree in the mist of the garden that was unclean and would harm them if they ate of it because he designed it that way. There was something in that fruit that contained a poison, however small it was. Maybe because of the way he designed our bodies or the earth, it wasn't good for us but it was good for the earth. When Eve ate of the fruit it caused an instant chain reaction that has lasted even until today.

We really can't be upset with Eve. Every day we put things in our bodies we know we shouldn't. Some of you smoke and know your wouldn't. Some eat certain candy bars and know how shouldn't; let me attempt to explain what happened in the Garden of Eden. Let's say I'm Adam or Eve. If I'm invincible that means nothing can hurt me. I've got all the food could want. I've got a beautiful mate by my side. I've got nothing to worry about. I mean Adam and Eve had to be some really great looking people. They were God's first creations. To my wife, Adam must have looked like Denzel Washington or Brad Pitt and for me Eve must be somewhere between Angelina Jolie and Janet Jackson –Have you seen Janet lately? In the beginning there was no fussing or fight-in. No one was going to die any time soon, in fact, not ever. There were no bills, no sickness, no work. We were chilling in Tahiti Baby. We shouldn't be worried about anything at all. I really shouldn't be worried about what I don't know. But, if Eve was anything like my first girlfriend, not know-in something was worse than death. So when the serpent said to Eve, "Don't you want to be all-knowing like God?" It was like a caffeine rush to Eve... "Each."

So, Eve takes a bite of the fruit, and instantly, in Eve's mind, a rush of knowledge over took her. She wasn't quite clear what it was because the most severe harm could not fall on her. The Bible says that the unbelieving spouse is covered by the believer. Eve then takes the fruit to Adam and he takes bite, also. As the Bible said, (Genesis 3:6-7):

6 And when the woman saw that the tree was good for food, and that it was pleasant to the eyes, and a tree to be desired to make one wise, she took of the fruit thereof, and did eat, and gave also unto her husband with her; and he did eat.

7 And the eyes of them both were opened, and they knew that they were naked; and they sewed fig leaves together, and made themselves aprons. "

Then it became crystal clear, they were going to die.

NOW they had something to worry about!

Like Superman and Kryptonite, one second He was invincible and the next second he felt weak. The first thought that crossed their minds was, "Will I die today or next Friday?" "Am I going to get sick?" "How do I protect myself?"

Maybe they thought, "I better put on some clothes this cold air doesn't feel so good anymore" because in verse 8 it says:

8 And they heard the voice of the LORD God walking in the garden in the cool of the day: and Adam and his wife hid themselves from the presence of the LORD God amongst the trees of the garden.

The minute this fruit, or this poison, entered their bodies..... Instantly, they knew the good times were over. That was the knowledge that God didn't think they needed to know. Before, they weren't ever going to die. THAT KNOWLEDGE WAS ON A NEED TO KNOW BASIS ONLY!

Have you ever heard of the "screen door effect?" If you place a bunch of dirt on a screen door and never clean it, eventually the dirt will get so thick that nothing will pass through the little holes not even water. But if you clean it and pour water on it – it goes right through it.

People can eat so many bad things that when one little bad thing enters their system, they don't even feel it.

Before I got into health food I could eat pizza, drink soft drink after soft drink and neither would have any effect on me immediately. When I got into health food, I cleansed my body with the program you'll read about later in this book. Now if I get little of anything that I shouldn't have, my body lets me know immediately. My diet is such now that when I eat a little sugar (sometimes even the natural turbinate sugar,) I can feel pain running down the arteries and veins in my arms, as the sugar molecules begin to solidify in my body.

Food Order and Body Clock

Build
8pm-4pm

Cleanse
4am-noon

Fruits
Protiens
Starches
No Dairy

Distribution
Noon-8pm

M&M Herbs

I make it a point not to eat processed sugar. If I were to drink a bottle of grape juice with sugar added to it, I can feel it within seconds. The something happens to me when I eat milk products. I can immediately feel mucus building up in my temples and nasal passages. Many people experience migraines this way.

We truly are what we eat. It's a profound statement, but a more profound one might be, "We are what we eat and what our parents and grandparents ate." Did you know what our ancestors ate can also have an effect in our bodies? The saying "the sins of the forefathers will be passed down seven generations" applies to the food laws in an awesome way.

Incest, drug use, and bad diets can cause horrible birth defects in children. Many blood diseases feel have a great deal to do with one of those three. The Bible says our body is the temple of God:

1 Corinthians 3:16 Don't you know that you yourselves are God's temple and that God's Spirit lives in you?

God didn't want us to get sick and die. Godhead designed our bodies in a fashion that we could live forever. If we simply didn't put certain toxins in our body it would have been possible. Unfortunately, that toxin was in the fruit that Adam and Eve ate. God warned us but we disobeyed. How many of us are still disobeying today? Because they disobeyed and we disobey we are still dying horrible deaths today. Some of you are saying, "What are we disobeying today?" Well, hold your horses. Let me finish the story. God banished them from the Garden, but just before he tells them to go he hands down the punishment. Three key things:

Genesis 3:15-1 9 Woman shall have great pain or sorrow in giving birth. Her desire shall be for her husband and he shall rule over her. Cursed is the ground for thy sake and in sorrow thou shall eat of it. And thou must work the landfill you sweat and eat the herb and make bread.

That was over 50,000 years ago. Not much has changed. Women still have pain in childbirth. In most countries a woman is still defined by her husband, who in those cases just happens to rule over her. And third, we still eat bread at just about every meal with some sort of herb or vegetable that was grown in soil that someone had to till and work.

Before the original sin, all we had to do was pick fruits in the garden and eat them. Now we would have to work hard to eat.

Let me make another statement. Since that time, we have been trying to change all of these things. We have C-sections and epidurals for birth-in. We have Hillary Clinton and Jane Fonda forth women's rights movement. We have man made foods and all kinds of machinery designed for the sole purpose of making the whole planting and plowing thing easier. All of these efforts either fall short or will eventually fall short of their expectations. Trust me people, we've been trying for over 50, 000 years. C-sections and epidurals both have their downfalls because of the possible complications and the pain after the procedure.

Some of you women are sitting there saying, "I don't need a man and a man will never rule over me." I have one thing to say about that. Every man knows that pound for pound, inch for inch that women are smarter and more intelligent than men. Women are very complex creatures; some may even be clairvoyant. Men are very simple creatures and don't need much, just a little attention here and there. Women operate out of a series of emotions. Men operate off of one emotion— His ego. Therein lies the root of the problem. The economic and social makeup of the world society will never be able to withstand women's control or equality. Why? Because men need to feel powerful to survive and the only time they can give genuine emotional support to a woman is when he feels powerful and his ego is being stroked. The smartest women in the world rule by "Honey do's" and that's in every culture. However, that's another book. I'll be happy to write about it some other time.

The topic that is most significant to us even today is that we're still trying to find ways to keep from plowing the soil and eating the herbs as they grow out of the earth. In Leviticus 25:1-5, God gives us laws for planting and growing.

"For six years sow your fields, and for six years prune your vineyards and gather their crops.4 but in the seventh year the land is to have a Sabbath of rest, a Sabbath to the LORD. Do not sow your fields or prune your vineyards. 5 Do not reap what grows of itself or harvest the grapes of your untended vines. The land is to have a year of rest."

These are laws that are followed by true organic farms and cultures where its citizens live long healthy vibrant lives but nowhere else.

Land Deficiencies

Today because of the rapid acceleration of the population and poor economic conditions for farmers, the plight is to produce as much food as possible and thereby never giving the land time to rest. We use pesticides, fertilizers and treated water to force the land into yielding a harvest. However, despite these efforts, God's laws still stand firm and unchanged.

In 1936, the Cosmopolitan Magazine published an article contained the following:

"Most of us today are suffering from certain dangerous diet deficiencies. The alarming fact is that foods -fruits and vegetables and grains - are now being raised on millions of acres of land that no longer contain enough of certain needed minerals. No matter how much of them we eat, these foods are starving us! Its bad news to learn from our leading authorities that 99 percent of the North American people are deficient in (vital)minerals, and that a marked deficiency in any of the more important minerals actually results in disease. "This article was based on the

findings that were listed in the 1936 US Senate bill #264 Which stated: "No man of today can eat enough fruits and vegetables to supply his stomach with the mineral salts he requires ..." Many states show marked reduction in the productive capacity of the soil...in many districts amounting to a 25 to50 percent reduction in the last 50 years... Some areas show a tenfold variation in calcium. Somehow a sixty-fold variation in phosphorous...Authorities... see soil depletion, barren livestock, increased human death rate due to heart disease, deformities, arthritis, increased dental caries, allude to lack of essential minerals in plant foods."

That was 1936. Today we are concerned to see the desert expanding to lands which only yesterday were prosperous and fertile. We are, for the most part, the cause of the barrenness of the lands which have become desert, just as we caused the pollution of the oceans and ground waters.

When we do not respect the goods of the earth, and abuse it, we are performing what I believe are criminal acts. Because of what we have done wearing poverty and death to those who follow in life after us.

In November 2006 WBZ in Boston ran a report about an article in the Journal of Science that said scientists believe by the year 2048 the ocean will not be able to support our eating habits because of overfishing. It said that many species will simply be unfindable because the population will be so small.

Pope John Paul II had this to say:

"We are deeply worried to see that entire peoples, millions of human beings, have been reduced to destitution and are suffering from hunger and disease because they lack drinking water. In fact, hunger and many diseases are closely linked to drought and water pollution. In places where rain is rare or the sources of water dry up, life becomes more fragile; it fades away tithe point of disappearing. Immense areas of Africa are experiencing this scourge, but it is also presenting certain areas of Latin America and Australia. - LENT 1993."

In 2002, the world grain harvest of 1,807 million tons fell short of world grain consumption by100 million tons, or 5 percent. The shortfall was the largest on record and marked the third consecutive year of grain deficits. Grain reserves then were at their lowest level in a generation and it hasn't got-ten any better. Still worse, farmers continue to plow highly erodible land that became that way due to over plowing. This land is too dry or too steeply sloping to sustain cultivation and can't possibly satisfy the increasing demand.

Each year billions of tons of topsoil are being blown away in dust storms or washed away in rain-storms, leaving farmers struggling to grow food foursome 70 million additional people with less topsoil than the previous year.

What happens to land when topsoil blows away? All you have to do is look in Ethiopia, Iraq and much of China. All of these places used to be fertile and full of abundant food but because of greediness and unwillingness to follow God's laws their land has turned to desert. In fact deserts are appearing all over.

In an article entitled "Sands of Time: Earth's Expanding Deserts Can't Be Stopped," published by the Pacific News Service, Commentary, Franz Schurmann, Apr. 06, 2005 SAN FRANCISCO— Instates that:

Dust storms and drought don't get as much press as hurricanes or rising sea levels, but they threaten the world nonetheless. They could even hit the 2008 Olympics in Beijing. On every continent the number of dust storms is increasing. The U.S. Department of Agriculture — once the second-largest bureaucracy in

Washington next tithe Pentagon, until Homeland Security bumped it— is not yet ready to proclaim a "Dust Bowl II."But it has released photos that show the awesome similarity between the first and the putative second dust bowl. Besides afflicting people with sundry diseases, dust bowls can ravage entire agricultural economies. The Dust Bowl of the 1930's forced thousands of "Okies" and "Aries" to immigrate to California. And Chinese environmentalists have raised the alarm after a survey earlier this year found almost a third of China's land mass is now desert.

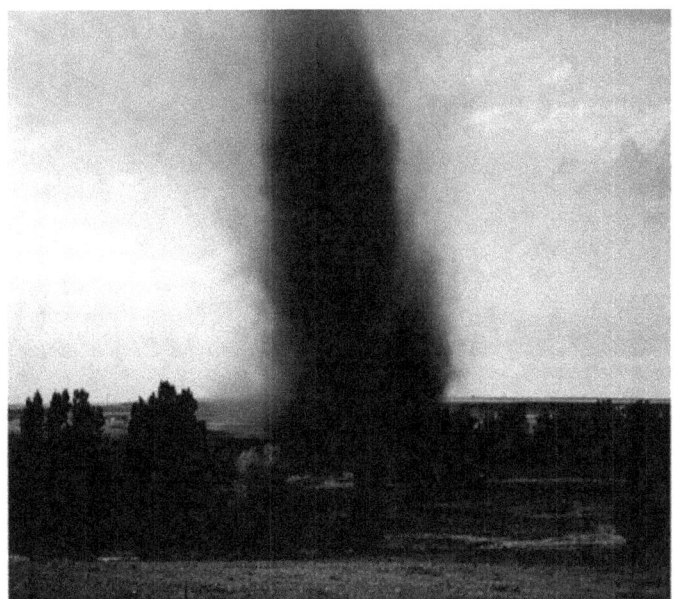

If you are next to an internet connected com-putter go to www.rainbowdiet.org *and search for a clip called "twister" and play it. You'll understand.*

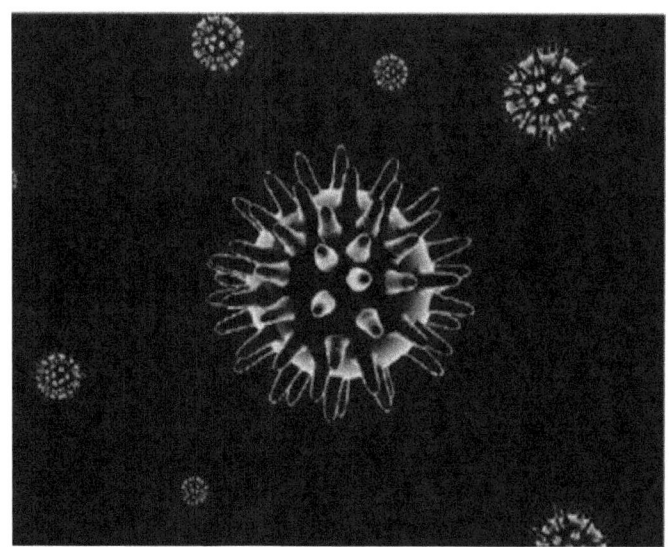

According to The Globalist magazine in March 12, 2004 Lester Brown wrote an article shrinking farmland:

The fall in China's grain harvest is due largely to shrinkage of the grain-harvested area from 90 million hectares in 1998 to 76 million hectares in 2003. Several trends are converging to reduce the grain area, including the loss of irrigation water, desert expansion, the conversion of cropland to nonfarm uses, the shift to higher-value crops and a decline in double-cropping. The last development is due to the loss of farm labor in the more prosperous coastal provinces, as farmers seek higher paying jobs elsewhere in the booming economy.

Chinese agriculturalists believe the reason they can't feed everyone in China is because they don't have enough labor to pull a second crop from the soil each year. The farmers in China are a lot smarter than this journalist thinks. Chinese farmers are getting going while the going is good because they know double cropping is not good for the land. They know the desert is expanding and that their land is yielding smaller and smaller crops. God's laws are awesome and unchanging. No matter how we try to change what he has put in place, his laws will win out in the end.

Elmer Josephson once made this statement:

There is no portion of the commandments of God in general, or of the Mosaic code in particular, that is not based on a scientific understanding of fundamental law. The laws of God are enforced and are as sure as his law of Gravity. You know the one Newton takes credit for.

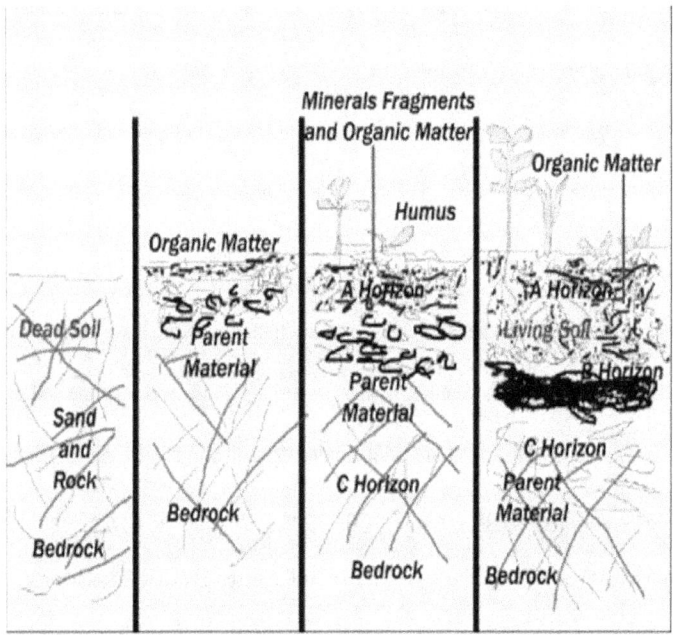

Let me attempt to explain soil and what makes it fertile. One square foot of fertile soil contains algae, fungi, billions of magical bacteria, as well as worms and other creatures each playing their important role in fertile soil. Each organism does its parting breaking down minerals that are large enough to see with the human eye into water-soluble molecules plants can absorb into their roots. When small floods occur during rainstorms and small deposits of silt are deposited on lower plains, the plants can do nothing with them. The organisms that live in the soil come to the rescue. The bacteria in the soil begin to break down the mineral deposits. Next the earthworms and beetles eat away at both the bacteria and the minerals. Their digestive tracts then breathe particles down farther and they excrete them out into even smaller forms that are absorbable by the plants. Also, the worms and beetles carry these minerals deep into the earth while burrowing tunnels in the soil- these tunnels act as storage containers for air and water in the soil.

The organic oils given off by the worms' bodies lubricate the tunnels and lock in moisture for small amounts of time. The more bacteria, worm and insect activity, the better the soil will be. Healthy land even builds its own defense system against disease and unwanted predators.

Overflowing tends to dishevel the small ecosystems in these soils. It is suggested that every seven years, one should allow the land to rest to give the organisms that live in it time to multiply and do their work without disturbance.

When we force the land to give crops continuously, it never gets to rest and the bacteria in the soil aren't strong enough to fight off the different diseases and larger insects that come to destroy crops. When this happens, we get angry and spray pesticides to get rid of the bugs that eat away at the crops, not realizing that we are killing the smaller organisms that live within the soil- the same organisms that are responsible for keeping it fertile in the first place. After we've killed off the soils inhabitants, we start to realize that the soil isn't as fertile as it was before, so we begin to add fertilizer. However, for the most part fertilizer is comprised of NPK (nitrogen, phosphorus and potassium) the three minerals plants need to grow and look good in appearance.

Most farmers seem to just forget about the other 87 plus minerals that should be included. It's kind of like feeding your child so he can grow to become an adult but never sending him to schools he can learn and be intelligent. The child would be robbed of being able to contribute to society; it's basically an empty shell. This is the same thing that happens to the soil. Deep fertile soil now becomes shallow because the soil's insects and organisms are not around to push the mineral nutrients deep into the soil.

Have you ever seen an anthill (mound)? Whatnot see on top of the soil is really just the tip of the iceberg. Underneath the soil is a much more extensive tunnel system that allows ants to store organic food matter deep in the earth. Ants are one of the few soil inhabitants that build their home in this split level way. There are literally millions of other organisms beneath the earth. All of the other inhabitant's homes extend deep into the soil and there is a constant cycle of matter being shuffled around in the soil. When we exterminate these inhabitant's the soil slowly loses its depth due topsoil runoff; as a result of the soil not being able to reproduce itself, the plant roots can only travel into the soil so far before they hit impenetrable bedrock or infertile nutrient lacking earth.

A similar thing happens when we use fertilizers. The plant roots don't need to go far to find the NPK because it's placed at the top of the soil by humans. Plants are what hold the topsoil's together. The inhabitants leave fecal matter and other slimy residue behind which all contain tiny deposits of water. This water is temporarily stored inside these deposits. Without them, the water will eventually wash away the plants with the shallow soil overtime revealing the bedrock underneath which is better known as desert sand.

If we don't start following God's laws we're doomed. The absence or chemical perversion of each of those other minerals is responsible for 100% of the sickness and disease that we go to our doctors to fix. We should go to the farmers with our problems. However, the average farmer doesn't care about our health. Most farmers are too busy trying to turn a profit to be concerned with the vitamin fortitude of their crop or the lack thereof.

Our Food Is Starving Us

Why are farmers not making good profits? First - they have to compete with foreign countries where labor is cheaper. Second - Mega farms are yielding more unhealthy food per acre and are able to offer better prices to grocery chains and food processors. Third- the land the farmers have is becoming unusable so they have to buy more. Four - they are competing with food substitutes and concentrated forms of their own products that are stored for longer periods of time.

Visit any grocery store and tell me how many items on the shelf are one hundred percent natural. That's where every ingredient on the label is water ores something that has not been processed in anyway except by squeezing (like juice) or chopping (like pineapple cubes.) It can't have any chemical com-pounds such as sodium benzoate or Acesulfame Po-passim or a natural substance that has been altered such as high fructose sugar, which has been subjected to extreme heat. (In many cases it has been bleached to hide impurities.) If you find one hundred out of the more than five thousand products (excluding the fruit and vegetable aisle,) I'd be surprised. Then find out how many are at least seventy-five percent natural. This number may still amaze you. A bottle of Enfamil baby food should frighten you. The fact is that short of the dry goods and the fresh goods aisle, most things are more than fifty percent man-made and have little or no nutritional value. Many of these man-made products cause some type of adverse affect on your body.

Most of us have an innate feeling that almost everything that is man-made is not good for us. We tell our kids not to eat junk food. We steer ourselves toward foods that say low fat, low sodium, or no trans fats. Even when we tend to go on binges and eat nothing but junk food our bodies begin to ache and weaken in an attempt to tell us we're doing the wrong thing. So why do we eat those man-made things in the first place? Because they taste so good! There's nothing like a twinkie or a cupcake but the truth is if you stuck one of those on a tool shelf outside in your garage they would still be there two hundred years later. No parasite or insect - not even mice will eat it because it's composition is almost entirely artificial.

All of these unhealthy things taste great but the things that are best for us are bland and have strange textures. For the most part, we don't haves miles on our face when we eat them in their original forms. The truth is most of us have sorrow when we have to eat beans and other vegetables in near natural form. I don't think anyone will argue that a snickers bar tastes better than string beans. No matter what we do the punishment God gave man for disobeying him will hold true. It will be only by his grace that any of us escape them, but we have to stop disobeying the laws that he has sat forth. In Leviticus, God gave us pretty detailed laws about

what is good for us to eat and what is bad for us to eat.

(Leviticus 17) It shall be a perpetual statute fory our generations throughout

ally our dwellings, that ye eat neither fat nor blood.

2 Speak unto the children of Israel, saying, these are the beasts which ye shall eat among all the beasts that are on the earth.

3 Whatsoever parteth the hoof, and is cloven-footed, and cheweth the cud, among the beasts, that shall ye eat.

4 Nevertheless these shall ye not eat of them that chew the cud, or of them that divide the hoof: as the camel, because he cheweth the cud, but divideth not the hoof; he is unclean unto you.

5 And the coney, because he cheweth the cud, but divideth not the hoof; he is unclean unto you. 6And the hare, because he cheweth the cud, but divideth not the hoof; he is unclean unto you.

7And the swine, though he divide the hoof, and be cloven-footed, yet he cheweth not the cud; he is unclean to you.

8 Of their flesh shall ye not eat, and their carcase shall ye not touch; they are unclean to you.

9 These shall ye eat of all that are in the waters: whatsoever hath fins and scales in the waters, in the seas, and in the rivers, them shall ye eat.

10 And all that have not fins and scales in the seas, and in the rivers, of all that move in thewaters, and of any living thing which is in the waters, they shall be an abomination unto you:

11They shall be even an abomination unto you; ye shall not eat of their flesh, but ye shall have their carcasses in abomination.

12 Whatsoever hath no fins nor scales in the waters, that shall be an abomination unto you.

Many of us eat swine (better known as pork.) Others eat seafood that don't have fins or scales (like shrimp, oysters or catfish.) A great deal of you don't know the difference between a catfish or a trout once it's on your plate. Have you ever cleaned or carved a fish? Can you tell the difference between a catfish and a trout? Just eighty years ago everyone who was of cooking age could tell you which fish had fins and gills and which did not because they were the ones who had to carve and clean the fish. We've separated ourselves from this entire process and have ignored these principles so much that we couldn't even get on the right track if we wanted too. We would need a teacher. Much of the blame belongs to misinformation or confusion, which is one of Satan's best tools.

1 Corinthians 14:33 For God is not the author of confusion, but of peace, as in all churches of the saints.

We as Christians have to hold fast to the Word. We should feel the same way about our food as we feel about abortion or child molestation. Instead we allow people to tell us things that are different and we believe them because it's what we want to hear.

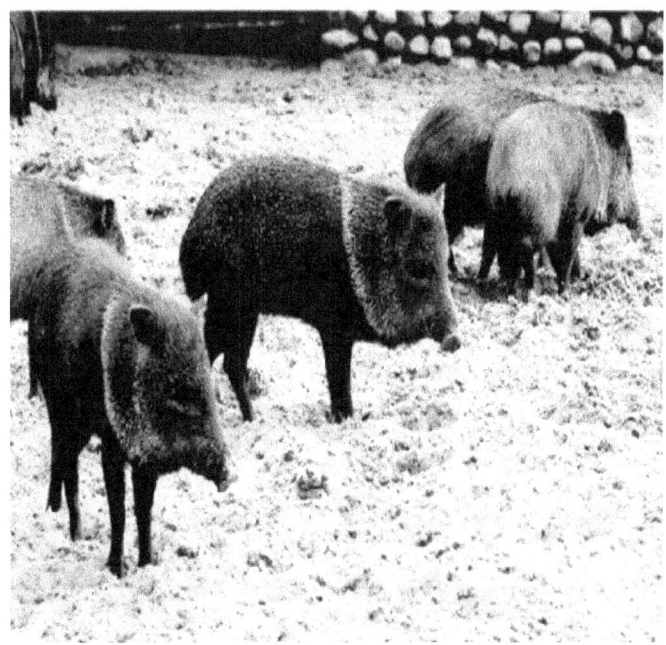

According to the CDC's website, a disease called trichinosis is caused by eating raw or under cooked meat of animals infected with the larvae of a species of worm parasites called Trichinella. Infection occurs commonly in certain wild carnivorous (meat-eating) animals but may also occur in domestic pigs. Pig's bodies contain MANYTOXINS, WORMS and LATENT DISEASES. Although some of these infestations are harbored in other animals, modern veterinarians say that pigs are far MORE PREDISPOSED to these illnesses than other animals. This could be because PIGS like to SCAVENGE and will eat ANY kind of food, INCLUDING dead insects, worms, rotting carcasses, excreta including their own, garbage,and other pigs. INFLUENZA (flu) is one of the MOST famous illnesses which pigs share with humans. This illness is harbored in the LUNGS of pigs during the summer months and tends to affect pigs and humans in the cooler months. Sausage contains particles of pig lungs and intestines.   Could this be a major source of human sickness?

An article ran in the Sunday, June 14, 2003 issue of the Baltimore entitled "China dinner delicacies succumb to SARS."

Some scientists theorized that SARS migrated from pigs to humans. A person can have various parasites like roundworm, pinworm, hookworm, etc. One of the most dangerous is Taenia Solium, which is in layman's terminology called tapeworm. It harbors in the intestine and is very long. Its ova (i.e. eggs,) enter the blood stream and can reach almost all the organs of the body. If it enters the brain, it can cause memory loss. If it en-ters the heart, it can cause a heart attack. If it enters the eye it can cause blindness. If it enters the liver, it can cause liver damage. It can damage almost all the organs of the body. A common misconception about pork is that if it is cooked well, these ova die. In a research project undertaken in America, it was found that out of twenty-four people suffering from Trichura Tichurasis, twenty two had cooked the pork very well. This indicates that the ova present in the pork do not die under normal cooking temperature. The Animal and Plant Health Risk Assessment Network and the Canadian Food Inspection Agency, located in Nepean, Ontario, Canada, said that: The animal health hazards associated with the importation of pork and pork products include four viral agents: foot and mouth disease, classical swine fever (hog cholera), African swine fever,and swine vesicular disease viruses.

In the United States, we have allowed people to tell us that its okay to eat unclean animals now because they are farm raised. Some ministers tell from the pulpit that God who is an unchanging God changed his mind and now these unclean foods are somehow not an abomination to our bodies. They use 1 Timothy 4:3, and Mark 7:19, as two of four source sin the Bible. When in fact 1 Timothy 4:3, if read carefully using the original Greek text says exactly the opposite and the latter part of Mark 7:19 which says, "Jesus did away with the law" is not even found in the original text. But first let's examine the King James Version of

1 Timothy 4:1 The Spirit clearly says that in later times some will abandon the faith and follow deceiving spirits and things taught by demons. 2 Such teachings come through hypocritical liars, whose conscience has been seared as with a hot iron. 3 They forbid people to marry and order them to abstain from certain foods, which God created to be received with thanksgiving by those who believe and who know the truth. (The Laws of Moses in Leviticus was the only thing he could have been speaking of when he said "truth.")

If you stop here its clear what is being said, however, if you read only the next verse by itself as so many pastors do, the meaning is cloudy, *Verse 4 For everything God created is good, and nothing is to be rejected if it is received with thanksgiving,* If you stop here or read only this verse in the King James version without the preceding context it can be deceiving. But if you read the fifth verse the true meaning becomes clear again.

Verse: 5 because it is consecrated by the word of God and prayer.

Even here the meaning is clear which says that if the "word" meaning "Moses' Law," consecrated it and if you pray over it then it is good. Some preachers seem to forget about the consecrated part of the verse and say if you pray for it then it is then "magically" good for you and is okay to eat. I am sometimes amazed at how easily pastors accept this notion. If this interpretation were correct it would mean that it would be okay for us to eat anything including a blow fish or any other organisms or plants that are considered poisonous. All we would have to do is simply pray over them. Still many preachers looking for an easy way out of the argument of a lifetime with their congregation ignore the context and only refer to verse 4. Take a closer look at verse 4 which is crystal clear in the Greek. Just like in the English language words can have similar meanings like "lost." If you say "I lost weight", you didn't really mean I lost it and I might stumble on it if I just look. It simply means it is gone. In the Greek "created" can mean, "Made" or it can mean "sanctified" or "sanctioned." In verse 4 the translation literally reads:

4 For everything which God has sanctified is good, and nothing is to be rejected if it is received with thanksgiving.

Now the verse no longer contradicts the other verses that surround it.

Take a look at Mark 7:15-19. It reads:

15 Nothing outside a man can make him 'unclean' by going into him. Rather, it is what comes out of a man that makes him 'unclean.'

16 If anyone has ears to hear, let him hear.

17 After he had left the crowd and entered the house, his disciples asked him about this parable.

18 "Are you so dull?" he asked. "Don't you see that nothing that enters a man from the outside can make him 'unclean'? 19 For it doesn't go into his heart but into his stomach, and then out of his body." (In saying this, Jesus declared all foods "clean.")

Notice that (In saying this, Jesus declared all foods "clean.") is in parenthesis ( ) marks. This is because that sentence doesn't exist in the original manuscripts.

In fact the story isn't even addressing abolishing laws of God. It is simply saying that even though the food is unclean it doesn't make the man's heart unclean. All anyone has to do is read the entire chapter for the real meaning.

So many times I visit churches where the "sick and shut in" lists read like a roll of a classroom and more than seventy percent of the congregation is overweight. How can we as Christians be an example to others if we're always getting sick? Would anyone listen to a minister if he's always coughing throughout the sermon and having to stop his sermon to go to the bathroom because he has a weak bladder? Why are there so many sick people in church? It is time to reclaim the health of our church people.

One Sunday I was in a service at First Baptist in Atlanta where Charles Stanley is the Pastor. He made a startling announcement. He said that months back he read Jordan Rubin's book The Makers Diet. The book expresses many of the same things you are reading in this book. As a direct result of Pastor Stanley's reading the book, he changed the menu in the church cafeteria to meet the requirements of the book. Months later the overall health of the staff had improved greatly. The PROOF was in a massive decrease in sick days taken and less claims on the church health insurance plan. As a result, at the end of the service Jordan and Pastor Stanley gave everyone in the audience a free copy of The Makers Diet; a twenty dollar book. There were over a thousand people at that service. Do the math - that was over $20,000 worth of books. I'd say someone was convinced!

Christians, we can't ignore the truth anymore. We now know that we should have been following the Old Testament diet all along just like our friends; the devout Jews, Muslims and very small Christian groups have done for thousands of years. All of these groups are strict eaters. They each have strict interpretations of God's food laws. For example;

Exodus 34:26 reads, "Bring the best of the first fruits of your soil to the house of the LORD your God. "Do not cook a young goat in its mother's milk."

My Jewish friends not only follow this principle but they don't eat anything that combines meat with dairy products such as pizza, ham and cheese sandwiches or cheese burgers. At the local Jewish summer camp where I help out and serves a camp counselor we are not even permitted to bring certain types of foods on the premises for fear that someone child may eat something they were not suppose to eat.

Muslims are not permitted to be in the same room with pork or other forbidden foods like alcohol. It's time that all of us begin taking note and be just as skeptical about what we eat and where we eat as they are. Many of us ask, "Why can't we eat milk with meat? Why not eat pork, why do this or that?" The Bible doesn't give a scientific study on why or why not. It simply says don't do it.

Every year science uncovers facts that prove the stories in the bible are true and that God's laws have good reasoning. The Bible says don't eat crustaceans like shrimp and oysters because they don't have fins and scales. [Recently, science has found that crustaceans because they have high levels of fat can absorb toxins out of the water at a much higher rate than other kinds of fish.] Because of this scientists now use crustaceans to test the concentration levels of mercury and lead pollution in the water. That means if we eat a crustacean we are putting those same toxins in our bodies.

Both the land and the ocean are inhabited by similar critters whose primary reason for living is to eat all the pollution that ends up in our environment. In the ocean, they are called "bottom feeders." On land, they are called rodents or scavengers. No matter what their name is we have harvested great amounts of these "environment cleaning" organisms and have turned them into food. Not only are we eating these toxins when we eat these organisms, but because we have taken so many of them out of their original homes, the land and the ocean can no longer clean themselves of the waste that poses huge threats to its other living inhabitants (i.e. you and me and the clean fish in the sea.)

Recently, animals that normally would not have toxins in them are being found with small levels of toxins. Clean fish like salmon and tuna are showing up positive with many of these toxins. Thankfully, almost all of the toxins are being found in the fatty tissue of these animals; the skin, the gut and the blood. The tissue God tells us not to eat. (Remember Leviticus...) If we don't eat those parts of the fish, we are generally safe. Moses Lived to 120. God created our bodies and the ecosystem to work in a perfect synchronized way. Even though we will all eventually die God created our bodies to live well past a hundred years and when we die we aren't supposed to be crippled and frail, begging to die because of a sickness that makes us suffer for months and years. Death should be quick and painless. The stories after we die should sound like" he went to sleep last night as happy as always but he didn't wake up this morning."

Deuteronomy 34:7 says, "And Moses was an hundred and twenty years old when he died: his eye was not dim, nor his natural force abated."

If we do what God says we will live long happy   prosperous lives. In the United States it's rare to see someone live past the age of one hundred. Of those who do, only a handful make it to one hundred and tenor more. In fact, in December 2004, Betty Wilson was the oldest person in America at 114 years old.

On that day Ms. Wilson day gained that illustrious title because Verona Johnston, who was born just a few months before her died at the same age.

Verona's daughter Julie says "She just wore out she was still very sharp until just a few months ago."

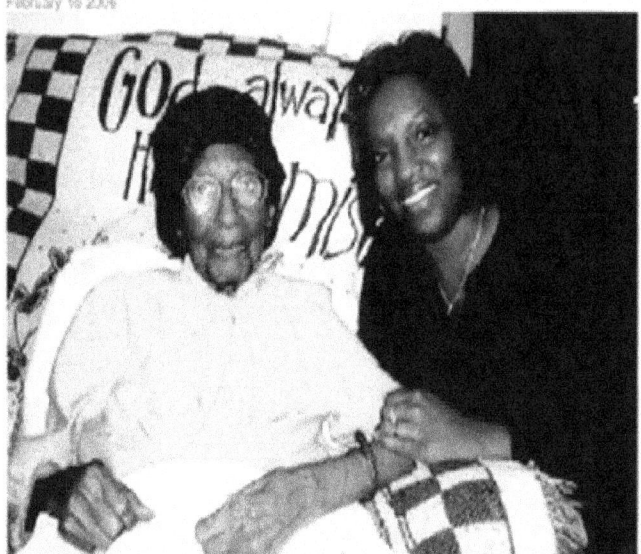

Bettie Wilson, the daughter of freed slaves who was one of the three oldest people in Am died Monday at her home in New Albany, Miss., of complications from congestive heart f according to her great-granddaughter Della Shorter. Wilson was 115.

Three people, all women, celebrated their 115th birthdays last summer.

Verona had voted in every election since 1920when women gained the right to vote. In the January1973 edition of National Geographic, a medical doctor named Alexander Leaf wrote an article on the oldest people in the world. On page 93 is a picture of a little lady smoking a cigarette. The caption next to the picture read:

"Serene at the summit of a long life." Kafaf Lasuira was more than 130 years old watches the world from the porch of her home in the then Soviet Union Abakhazia an autonomous Republic of Georgian SSR. She was nudged into retirement from her job as a tea leaf picker two years earlier... that did not stop her. She was still active around the house at 130 years old. By today's governing principles, she could have retired twice. Can you imagine the amount of social security she would have accumulated during that time? Not only that, Mrs. Lasuria likes to start her day off with a little fun.

The article reads on to say,

"Mrs. Lasuria enjoys a little vodka before breakfast and her daily pack of cigarettes."

I'm not advocating smoking cigarettes or drinking, but it is important to note that the Bible says it's okay to have a little drink here and there.

1 Timothy 5:23 Stop drinking only water, and use a little wine because of your stomach and your frequent illnesses.

There is much debate over was this wine fermented (containing alcohol) or not. However   science has recently found that a substance found in both, Resveratrol fights disease & extends life.

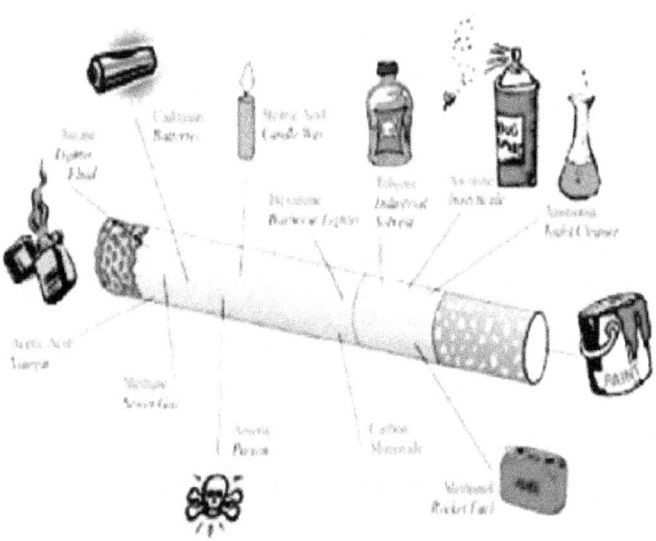

The worst thing about smoking a cigarette is not smoking the tobacco, but smoking the pesticides that were placed on the tobacco before it was harvested and chemicals contained in the paper.   Cadmium, mercury, lead and other toxic chemicals when burned produce poisonous gases that can kill those who breathe it first or second hand. A few pages over in the National Geographic article you'll see an old gentleman taking an odd looking bath. He's 104 year Markiti Tarkill. The caption beside his picture is a quote from Dr. Leaf.

"I was so amazed at such exertion by a man over a hundred. But wherever I went the level of physical activity among such old people was high."

On page 10311 7 year old Gabriel Chapnian carries a pail of newly harvested potatoes home for lunch up an Abkhazain hill that exhausted the author. The lifelong farmer continues to work half a day in the fields. - His prescription for longevity - "Active physical work, and a moderate interest in alcohol and the ladies." (Note here that the keyword is moderate; too much of either one will kill you, especially at that age)

For all you single guys that wonder when is the right age to get married and settle down. You might want to take note of Shirali Mislimov who is the guy on the next page of the article and was born in1805. That made him 168 years old at the time the article was written. At that time he was still riding horseback and tended "to the orchard which he planted in the 1870's."

Mislimov said that he married his 120 – year old wife 102 years ago. That means for those of you who aren't gifted in math, at the age of 66 he married an 18 year old girl. Unfortunately, Mr. Mislimov died a few months after this article was published, but he is considered to be the oldest man to have lived in recent times who had any kind of documentation. There are people who have claimed to have been older but their documentation was very vague and unreliable. Frankly, before the 1800'salmost no one had documentation of their birth unless they lived in a well educated or advanced village. However, this is not the focus of my message.

All of these people had a few things in common. The first of which was that they were all still in good health up until a few months before their death. If you look further in that article, you'll find even more things in common.

On Page 110 of the article Dr. Leaf says:

"Whether slim or not, the old people of all three cultures share a great deal of physical activity. The traditional farming and household practices demand heavy work, and male and female are all involved from early childhood to terminal days. Simply crossing the hills by foot during the day's activities sustained a high degree of cardiovascular fitness as well as general muscle tone."

Wow! Wouldn't you like to be cardio fit and muscle toned at 120?

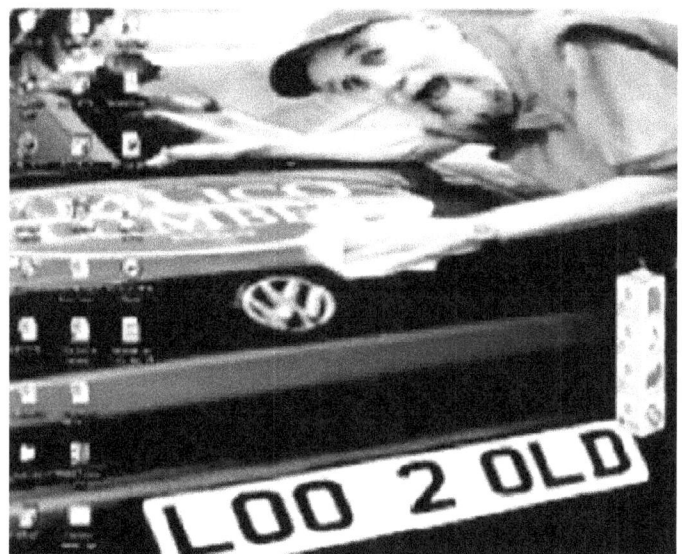

A man I greatly admire is "Buster" Martin who was forced into retirement at age 100. In fact, I use his picture as a screensaver on my laptop. You see - at 100, he was still working as an auto mechanic in Great Britain. It takes a good deal of strength and brain power to work on automobiles. Have you ever tried to unscrew a lug nut or figure out what part of your car needed to be worked on by just listening to the engine? So, you know it's no easy task. Can you imagine doing this at 100 years old? All of my research has shown that it is important to remain physically active every day of your life. Buster's secret is: He's never owned a phone in his life. He says phones keep him from "working peacefully." If you love what you do, working is not a bad thing. In fact, on page 113 of the National Geo-graphic Magazine, Dr. Leaf says,

"There is also a sense of usefulness. Even those well over 100 for the most part continue to perform essential duties and contribute to the economy of the community. These duties included weeding in the fields, feeding the poultry, tending flocks, picking tea, washing the laundry, cleaning house, or caring for grandchildren and in some cases great great grandchildren all on a regular basis."

Another key thing these centurions all had in common was the fact that most have had very little contact with doctors for medical purposes. Some-thing that should also be considered is that all were heterosexuals and most were married or had been. On page 112 Dr. Leaf references a colleague of his, Professor Pitzhelauri, who had collected figures relating marital status to longevity. He found from studies of 15,000 persons older than 80 that, with rare exceptions, only married couples attain extreme age. Many couples had been married 70, 80, or even 100 years. He concluded that marriage and a regular prolonged sex life are very important to longevity. USA Today published an article in2005 from The National Center for Health Statistics. It showed similar findings. The study included 127, 545 adults and said that married people were in general more healthy than singled people.

Dr. Leaf also says women who have many children tend to live longer. His figures showed that among the centenarians only 2.5 percent of the marriages were childless, whereas forty-four percent of the women had four to six children; twenty-three percent had only two or three; and nineteen percent had ten to fifteen. Several had more than twenty children. Buster has 17 children and 70 grandchildren and he married when he was 14 years old. Have you heard people say children keep you young? Many of the women had children well after age fifty; which you should know that this is not an uncommon thing.

Aleta James of New York understands. At age56, she delivered not one but two children - yes, twins. In 2005, a Romanian woman gave birth to a baby girl at 66 years of age. Yet again, in August 2006 in Great Britain, a vibrant 63 year old woman gave birth. They're not the only ones.

There are stories of 75 to 100 year old men impregnating their younger wives, more recently The great actor Tony Randall, known for his role in the TV sitcom "The Odd Couple," impregnated his 29 year old wife twice after age 77. So for those of you wanting to increase your life expectancy, pull out those old Nat King Cole records and get busy.

Eating Habits Matter

Dr. Leaf found many other similarities between the people he studied: diet wise meat and dairy products constituted very low parts of their diets. In three of the cultures they were only one and a half percent of their diet. Almost all dairy products were goat products and not from cows. These people grew all of their own food and didn't depend on someone else to grow it for them. Vegetables were the largest parts of their diets. Dr. Leaf found no signs of malnutrition in any of these cultures.

In contrast to the centurions, in the U.S. and Europe we have much higher divorce rates. It is now over 50%. On average we have 2.5children. We strive to retire at age 65 or earlier and homosexuality is common.

Our diets are almost the exact opposite of the centurions. Malnutrition in our supposedly highly evolved country is running rampant. Obesity can be found in more than half the population. Calcium deficiency causes more than 200 different diseases in our culture. Among those are arthritis, tooth decay, hemorrhoids, varicose veins, osteoporosis and high blood pressure which are one of the most deadly.

In America alone some 10 million people have high blood pressure. Every year some 1,000,000 people die from strokes caused by high blood pressure. In these cultures where people traditionally live past 80 and near and above 100, there is no obesity, high blood pressure, osteoporosis, Arthritis, tooth decay and they don't "got milk."

In America the rainmen as I like to call them would lead you to believe that without milk you're going end up with calcium deficiency - when the exact opposite is more likely true. The United States and parts of Europe lead the world in calcium deficiency diseases; it just so happens that these countries also lead the world in cow's milk consumption. The truth is that for most people in the United States cow's milk is very hard to digest. In fact the only group of people that consistently possessed the enzymes needed to digest the casinate and lactose found in milk were Caucasian women between the ages of 15-35. Just over 65% of these women were found to have the enzyme. If you think about it in the context of school everyone else scored an "F" and this group only got a "D." In my house hold a "D" is not acceptable. African American and Mexican American Women scored the lowest.

Source Cornell University
:

Post Slashdot, del.icio.us, Digg,
to. Furl, Netscape, Newsvine,
reddit, Yahoo! MyWeb

Date: June 2, 2005

Lactose Intolerance Linked To Ancestral Environment

ITHACA, N.Y. -- Got milk? Many people couldn't care less because they can't digest it. A new Cornell University study finds that it is primarily people whose ancestors came from places where dairy herds could be raised safely and economically, such as in Europe, who have developed the ability to digest milk.

Evolutionary Biologist Paul Sherman of Cornell University published a study in June 2005 which stated that Asian-Americans, African-Americans and American-Indians many times had less than a ten percent tolerance to milk lactose.

The problem here is that people in these groups still eat these lactose dairy products. The immediate effect on them is constipation which usually goes unnoticed due to published misinformation, put out by the rainmen that says it's okay to have a bowel movement once or twice a week. These same people begin to gain weight and lose all resemblances of a waist line all caused by an expanding, compacted intestinal tracts. These people continue to eat these products and by the time they start seeing the worst effects of these products, (the cancers and other side effects of obesity like high blood pressure,) it's usually too late. Others have adverse reactions to lactose such as diarrhea and severe allergies. They know they can't eat these products and thus label themselves as lactose intolerant. What they should call themselves are "severe lactose intolerant," because the rest of those people out there who can't easily digest this protein are slowly killing themselves. When they can't digest this enzyme it prevents them from being able to digest many other things and thus damages the entire digestion process. This causes food particles to build up in their intestinal tract thus causing them to gain weight. The end result is that every meal they eat which contains dairy products will essentially sit in theirs stomach giving them very little or no nutritional benefit at all. It will not readily move through their digestive tract; it just sits there in the intestines.

Many times particles will sit there for months if not years, turning into harmful toxins.

Okay everyone, here is the moment you've been "weighting" for. In 1994, I weighed 205 pounds, 40 pounds overweight.

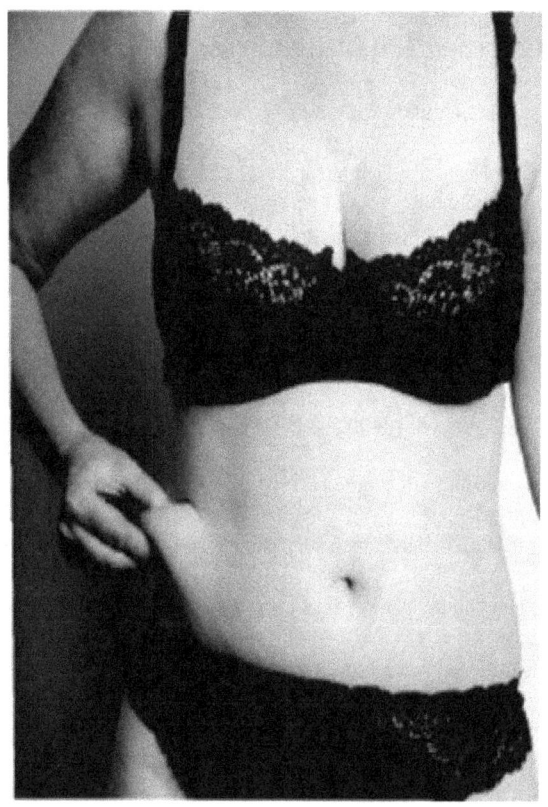

That year I discovered "My Body Clock" and what correct "Food Order" was. I lost 50 pounds in 6 months by simply changing the way I ate. I lost so much weight so fast that my grandmother swore I had HIV. However, the only thing that had occurred was digestive salvation.   Let me address this for a moment. The rainmen would lead you to believe that one or two bowel movements a week is okay, when in fact two or three bowel movements a day is healthy. The truth is that every time you eat a meal you should have bowel elimination within a few hours. When something goes in, something should come out (pushed out "if I may.")

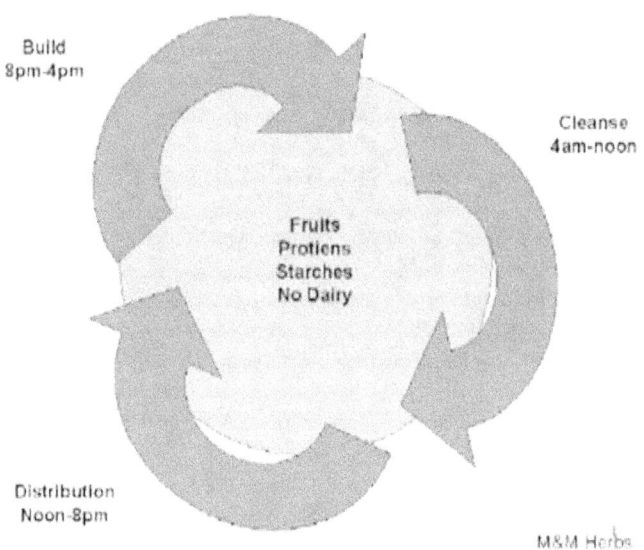

Food Order and Body Clock

Build
8pm-4pm

Cleanse
4am-noon

Fruits
Protiens
Starches
No Dairy

Distribution
Noon-8pm

M&M Herbs

Your body works on three basic cycles a day: Build, Cleanse, and Distribution. Each cycle requires fuel which is the food we eat which means that you should eat at least once during each cycle. If you eat less than that your body will respond in a number of different ways one of which is a camel like effect where the body stores food. Your body does this because it believes it's in danger of being starved. All of these effects will hinder your digestion thereby leaving you with less vitamins and minerals from an already mineral depleted food supply.

The food you eat during each cycle is important. During your "Cleanse cycle," which occurs between 4 am and 12 pm, it is important that you eat foods that are easily digestible. Fruit, when eaten by itself, digests in under 30 minutes, this means that you get the vitamins and minerals from them quickly. It's important that you get them into your body quickly each morning because you have just broken your nightly fast. You've usually just gone about 11 hours without eating, almost a half a day. This is why we call it breakfast. If you eat solid fruits by themselves in the morning, like an apple or a pear, you'll notice two things in a few hours following - one, you'll need to go to the bathroom and -two, you'll be hungry again.

Remember, eating an item from each fruit group by itself is essential in the digestive process. Everything else you eat takes three to four times as long to digest. If you combine fruit groups with anything else, it causes bloating as I will explain later.

Foods Groups

Starches	Protiens	Solid Fruits	Citrus Fruits	Melons	Dairy	Vegetables
Corn	Eggs	Apples	Oranges	Grapes	Milk	Greens
Pasta	Beef	Pears	Lemons	Plums	Cheese	Leeks
Bread	Seafood	Mangoes	Tangerines	Watermelons	Sour Cream	(Green) peas
Rice	(Brown) Beans				Ice Cream	Squash
Potatoes	Pork					Zuccini
Bananas	All Meats					Peppers
	Nuts					
	Coca Nut					

At lunchtime (launch-time), you start the distribution cycle (or the launching of needed materials throughout your body) which is your body's perfect time for taking in a medium to large sized meal. This is the best time to eat proteins by themselves or accompany them with vegetables. Proteins are the hardest thing for your body to break down so when you eat them, they should be eaten by themselves or with lightly cooked vegetables which still possess enzymes that will help you digest the proteins and the vegetables. A good way to prepare your body for proteins is to eat citrus fruits or drink organic non-concentrated orange juices about thirty minutes before this meal. Citrus fruits contain hydrochloric acid which is exactly the thing your digestive tract needs to breakdown proteins more effectively so you can get the most out of them.

Around 3:30 p.m. to 5:30 p.m. is always a great time for a nutrition bar to give you a little more boost as you near the end of the work day.

By dinner time you are nearing the Build cycle which is between 8 p.m. and 4 a.m. At night while you are sleeping your body assimilates the nutrients that you have appropriated during the day to the areas that need them. Whatever is not used is eliminated during your cleanse cycle the next morning.   Is this all starting to make sense to you now? God puts everything in perfect order. During the Build cycle your body needs the most energy. By now, your body is completing the most vital stage of breaking down the protein you ate at lunch. It is now ready for some powerful energy which you'll get out of the starches and vegetables in the next meal.

Be careful with your starches. The best ones are corn, baked potatoes and rice. Breads these days contain too many processed ingredients to provide much nutrition. In most cases unless you control the baking, I would highly recommend against it. However, if you are fortunate enough to find Ezekiel Bread or have a bread machine which you can make good bread in go ahead and eat it. Most of us have completed eating dinner by 8 p.m. That's okay, the food you ate between 6 p.m. and 8 p.m. will just be breaking down in time for the start of the Build cycle -that's only if you didn't mix anything in such as fruits or proteins. It's important that the starches be eaten with vegetables only because they require an alkaline enzyme to breakdown. Your body readily produces these when starches are eaten. In contrast when you eat a protein at the same time it tries to produce both hydrochloric acids and alkaline acids which are exactly opposite. If you remember back when you had chemistry in high school, those two substances negate each other. In a test-tube or flask, it is called "fizzling" or in severe cases - "an explosion." In our bodies we call it "gas," "belching," and in severe cases "heartburn."

No matter what you call it, when it's all said and done, it's simply indigestion and the worst thing you can add to this condition is an antacid which stops the digestion process all together. Once an antacid joins the digestive process, foods will run through your body at a slower pace and any chance of getting vitamins and minerals out of that meal is just about lost. Instead of taking an antacid when this occurs you should take something called a digestive enzyme (Food Enzymes.) Remember those are for the problem once it exists, but the best thing to do is to prevent indigestion from ever happening. It is very important not to mix proteins and starches! If you follow these instructions, your body will be free to move through the Build cycle while you sleep. From this point the cycle will start over again and the more you practice these principles the healthier you will be.

Great Kingdom, Weak Kingdom

This food order thing is very similar to what ancient cultures were eating before modernization. Even the centurions admit that when they were younger, their meals were more closely related to a diet like this one.

If you study the diets of non-modernized cultures that follow proper cultivation techniques and practice food ordering all over the world, you'll find that they have less disease and far better health. Most non-modernized countries and some modernized countries still follow these diet practices. French people, for example, have less body fat than Americans. Incidentally USA today featured an article in its January 4, 2005 edition called "The French Diet Connection" subtitled "Their Slimming Secrets- eating with sense." It featured an example of the typical French diet - which, by the way, did not include French fries. The lunch and dinner were perfectly combined; however, the breakfast ventured a little more toward the modernized diet.

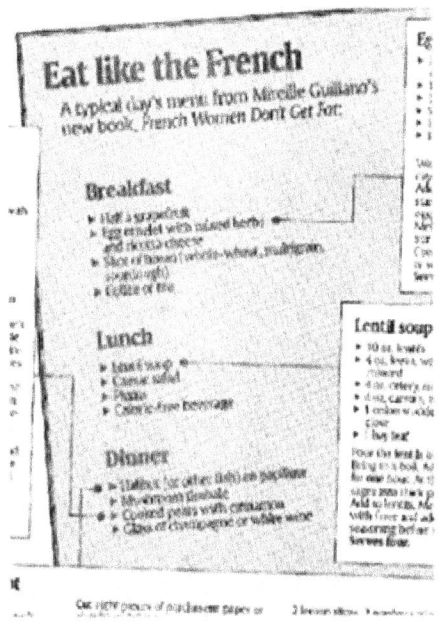

In 1913, a Nobel Prize – winning physician Albert Schweitzer visited Gabon, Africa which is one of the non-modernized countries which still follow proper eating habits. Gabon is located on the west side of the Congo near the coast. There, Dr. Schweitzer found no cases of cancer. He said "This absence of cancer seemed to be due to the difference in nutrition of the natives compared to the Europeans.   In the 1930's, a dentist from Harvard named Dr. Weston Price studied small villages populated by the Inuit Eskimo people of Canada, Australian aborigines, the New Zealand Maori and the Indians of South America. Ponce De Leon thought the fountain of youth must have existed in South America because of the healthy people of old age he found there.

A Nutritional Guide for Healing, Diet, and Well-Being
Tariq M. Sawandi, M.H., N.D.

As far back as 1913, Dr. Albert Schweitzer, the world famous medical missionary to Africa , discovered the basic cause of cancer. Although he had not isolated the specific nitriloside compound, he was convinced from his observations that a difference in food was the key. In his preface to Alexander Berglas's book, Cancer: Cause, and Cure, he wrote:

On my arrival in Gabon (Africa) in 1913, I was astonished to encounter no cases of cancer. I saw none among the natives two hundred miles from the coast....I cannot, of course, say positively that there was no cancer at all, but, like other frontier doctors, I can only say that, if any cases existed, they must have been quite rare. This absence of cancer seemed to be due to the difference in nutrition of the natives compared to the Europeans..."

From all over the African continent, the one thing Africans have in common is that the degree to which they are free from cancer is in direct proportion to the amount of nitriloside found in their diet. As much as 80% of the tropical African diet consists of nitriloside and thiocyanate yielding foods. The main staples of sub-Sahara Africa are cassava, yams, sorghum, and millet grains. Let us reinforce our knowledge with the science of how nitriloside foods work to fight cancer, sickle cell anemia and other chronic diseases.

Dr. Price and his wife realized that the diets of these non modernized people brought forth almost perfect teeth and that they had almost no tooth decay. Dr. Price found that the diets of these people contained much higher amounts of water soluble vitamins, and minerals - the most astounding one being calcium which was four times as much as those in the modernized world.

Their diets also contained ten times the fat soluble vitamins like A, D, and E. These just happen to be the same vitamins which a doctor by the name of T. Colin Campbell used in a study on cancer the first in 1983 and the second between1989 and 1990.

The name of Dr. Campbell's study is "The China Study." Dr. Campbell is now head of the nutritional sciences department at Cornell University in Ithaca, New York. He studied a unique tribe of people in China in that they ate the same thing every day of their lives and they rarely, if ever, left the village in which they grew up. The tribe was like having an earthly test tube. Dr. Campbell divided the villagers he chose for his experiment into three groups. The first he gave placebos, the second he gave only one of the vitamins and the third he gave all three vitamins. Out of his study came a great deal of information of which was published across the world. The project has been featured as a cover or lead story in numerous news print media, including USA Today, China Daily, and New York Times, among many others. The China Study was shown on television in Tokyo, Seoul, London, Frankfurt and the U.S. as part of documentaries.

"The dietary patterns in China are extremely different from Western countries, the major difference being the consumption of foods of animal origin. Animal protein intake for example, is 10-fold greater on average in the U.S. than in China. Although the biology of the diet and disease relationship is infinitely complex and is easily misunderstood when interpreted in a reductionism manner, the main nutritional conclusion from this study is the finding that the greater the consumption of a variety of good quality plant-based foods, the lower the risk of those diseases which are commonly found in western countries (ex., cancers, cardiovascular diseases, diabetes). Based on these and other data, we hypothesize that 80-90% of all such diseases could be prevented before about age 90 years."

THE
CHINA
STUDY

STARTLING IMPLICATIONS FOR DIET,
WEIGHT LOSS AND LONG-TERM HEALTH

T. COLIN CAMPBELL PhD
WITH THOMAS M. CAMPBELL II

The China Study
Author(s): T. Colin Campbell, Ph.D.
with Thomas M. Campbell
ISBN: 9321303865
Price: $24.95
Publication Month: January 2005
Publisher: BenBella Books
Hardcover

The suggestion that some countries are nutritionally better than others simply because of the practices they follow is not a new idea. When you look back in history, do you ever think about what made the great nations great and why did they eventually fall? The major reason the Egyptian culture gained so much fame and notoriety is because their agricultural practices were so far advanced when compared with other cultures. Their soil was considered the most fertile of all and because of this their "high quality food" was sought by men from all over the world. History shows that for thousands of years they enjoyed the benefits of great health evidenced by their great physical strength and stamina.

Near the end of the Egyptian's great era, practices began to change for the worst. From the consumption of pigs as food to poor and over-harvested land this is a common cycle in many civilizations. Once a generation approaches greatness and begins to get something right, their offspring usually forgets what it took to become a great civilization, disrespects their ancestors hard work by doing what at one point was highly practiced against usually in the name of having an easier more exiting life.

The Mayan Indian culture was another example. They met a similar demise. History says they were a great civilization that virtually destroyed itself and disappeared overnight.

When your food disappears or ceases to be nutritious, it doesn't take long for you to disappear. Either sickness sets in and you die, or you are forced to move on to a better place as fast as possible. The American Indians are another example. Bone samples of Indians who were around before modern agricultural practices began to set in show less bone disease than those who were afterward.   Civilization after civilization has risen and fallen around their agriculture practices. The bottom line is that big business doesn't matter. It doesn't matter how many cars or televisions you can make. If you don't have a strong base of natural nutritional resources your community will soon begin to lose its economical base and soon its existence.

The Ethiopian people you see depicted on television experiencing hunger pains are a perfect example of this. Ethiopia was once considered one of the most nutrient rich places on earth. Some even believe that it was once the location of the Garden of Eden. Centuries of incorrect agricultural practices have left a great deal of its people in a land that has now turned into a desert and can produce no food. A large majority of them now depend on the rest of the world to support them. Their society is dying off at an unbelievable rate. You've heard the stories right there on your Television. "Everyday thousands or more youth die of malnutrition and they need your help." I believe what they really need is an airlift out because the land is dead from over-harvesting and it will be dead for another thousand years or more. That's how long it will take before the land can repair itself and maybe once again become fertile.

Dr. Susan J. Herlin, a noted African researcher wrote this in her 2003 study of Ethiopia and surrounding areas: "the development of more efficient agriculture, larger settlements, and local competition over resources probably gave rise to early forms of warfare, that is, organized, violent conflict over territory, as walled villages in the Tichitt and Lake Chad areas testify." Also, a classic theme of human conflict was born when cattle herders and farmers of the northern savannas were faced with diminishing resources as the Saharan lands began to get progressively drier after 3,000 BCE. By about 2500 BCE basically modern climatic conditions existed in Africa north of the equator. A massive desert was growing from the banks of the Red Sea in the east to the Atlantic Ocean in the west, and from near the Mediterranean in the north to only a few hundred miles north of the present-day Sahel in the south. "Between 9000BC and 2500 BC. The Sahara which was once aquatic became a desert.

Study after study has been done, but still no widespread action. The problem is now so huge that no one person or group can change the pattern.

The Death of a Race

All my life I was taught to look at things for what they are and not to read too much into anything and don't believe all of the propaganda surrounding an issue. I am not politically correct by any means and I rarely hold my tongue. When I believe something needs to be said I usually say it. The next few paragraphs may get this book banned on shelves across America but if you will just hear me out I think you'll agree with me.

Take a look at this scenario. If you were standing in a McDonald's and a person walked in and began behaving like a dog, barking, walking around on all fours and asking for their coke to be poured into a bowl. What would you think? Would it be safe to assume that the person could be considered mentally ill? If the person was not being paid to pretend to be a dog and barring some sort of practical joke. The next logical assumption would be that this behavior was either chemically induced by some type of drug or this person was truly mentally ill and needed to be institutionalized. Now, let me add to this scenario. What if one in every five persons was behaving this way; including your governor and maybe even the mayor, and some lawyer who thought he was also a dog decided to pass a law which said, behaving like a dog was your natural right. What would you think?

Would the fact that there was a law which forbids you from doing something about the dog people alter your perception or attitude about the dog people? The answer to any logical person should be no, but in America and too many other countries unfortunately the answer is yes. Many of us have accepted those people with obvious chemically induced or mental issues as the norm and have simply decided not to do anything about it as the condition continues to spread amongst us. As I shop in the mall, eat in restaurants or drive around downtown every day I see men dressing like ladies behaving in ways that are stereotypical to women. Likewise, I see women dressing like men behaving in ways that are stereotypical to men. In recent months many states have passed bills legalizing same sex marriages. To some people I know, and much to my surprise, they are totally okay with this. They are totally okay with what I believe is a chemically induced behavior. A chemical found in plastic, a product since the 1960's which has slowly begun to take the place of glass and is now used in just about everything we eat or touch. The specific chemical is BPA (biphenol A.)

BPA disrupts any process that estrogen normally mediates, affecting brain, body, and behavior. The January 2012 edition of Psychology Today read like this "There is evidence that BPA emasculates males and makes them sexually undesirable to females.

"One of the prominent effects of early BPA exposure is that it eliminates a number of sex differences in brain and behavior," the researchers wrote. It turned out that BPA-exposed males have impaired spatial ability (can't find their way out of a maze or to their nest, considered unattractive to females). They also suffer from decreased exploratory ability (incurious and easily lost), and overall reduced attractiveness to the opposite sex. They may even smell different from their peers —in rodents, a sign of unhealthiness. Females are disgusted." The above findings were initially discovered by medical doctor David Feldman, a professor at Stanford University as early as 1992. In an experiment Feldman observed estrogen from yeast behaving differently in plastic flasks than in the glass flasks. He then did the test without the yeast and found that the plastic flasks were producing estrogen independent of yeast.

More test revealed that the chemical causing the estrogen like reactions was BPA a substance which is only banned in baby products but not in adult products. "Go figure!"

In society we call this phenomenon the gay agenda, the sexual revolution, the lgbt movement, and many other names but I ask you all to take a step back and look at it for what it really is – mass chemical exposure. The gradual build up and usage of this chemical and other hormones in our food supply has parralled the growth of homosexual activity in our society. Since 1960 worldly acceptance of this behavior has grown at a rate unlike any other time in history.

Many people I know whom happen to be homosexual say they feel u. These people need help. Folic acid and B12 are the only substances that havlike the other sex inside. I believe they are telling me the truth 100%. Just because they are telling the truth doesn't mean I am to accept it and neither should yoe proven effective in reversing the reactions of BPA. The simple truth to the matter is this. If homosexuality becomes the norm then eventually in the not so far future the population will seize to exist. We are heterosexual beings by nature not asexual or homosexual. It doesn't take a rocket scientist to see this.

Homosexuality is a sickness and should be classified as a disease!

The Revolution

We need a revolution. Yes, the term "revolution" falls under the category of "whatever it takes". What we have to do now is something like what Muslims call a "Jihad" or a "holy war". No not a GUNS AND WEAPONS war but an economic war. The Bible says money answers all things, but the love of money is the root of all evil. The love of money is the reason we have all of the health problems in the first place.

1 Timothy 6:10 For the love of money is a root of all kinds of evil.

Ecclesiastics 10:19 A feast is made for laughter, and wine makes life merry, but money is the answer for everything.

Farmers try to cut costs and raise profits by using fertilizers and pesticides. Pharmaceutical companies spend money on creating drugs, which they can patent for which they collect revenue, rather than spending money testing natural things such as herbs and sea plants. The automobile industry, for fear of losing tons of money in gasoline car sales, has done everything to halt the production of cars that run on clean fuels. Only the hybrid gasoline electric engines have been allowed to come on the market full steam, primarily because these vehicles able to please both the oil industry and the environmentally conscious worlds. Now look at the sales. These hybrid cars are some of the hottest selling cars on the road. It's called supply and demand and the customer runs the market. As consumers we must demanded change. The Atkin's Diet is one of the best examples of social health change I can think of. As a business consultant, I have consulted many restaurants. Once the Atkin's Diet began to become popular and was the in thing. Everyone was hopping on the Atkin's bandwagon; even schools were getting in to it. The food and restaurant industry felt the effects right away. The company which made Twinkies even filed for bankruptcy.

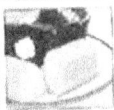
The Atkin's Diet told willful dieters everywhere to only eat proteins and cut out most starches, like bread. Dieters would go to restaurants and not eat any bread but they would ask for extra veggies or protein instead. Many restaurants died a slow painful death.

Most restaurants owners are very people oriented folks and they want to please their patrons. The majority I've come in contact with were mediocre businessmen at best and usually they don't read diets books. In fact they look at diets as something that is not favorable to their businesses.   For those of you who are not familiar with the Atkins Diet, the diet simply suggests that you should eat meals with protein only or with veggies but no high carbs like starches. This produced a slow undetectable issue with most restaurants. Most of restaurants simply put out bread on the table and never really ask you whether you would like bread or not. It's one of those collective reasoning things. Everyone else is doing it, so should we. Guests would go to the restaurants and not eat the bread. Instead they'd ask for extra veggies or proteins; when they got up from the table the bread basket would still be full and all of their potatoes were still on their plate.

Whenever a struggling restaurant calls me for help the first thing I say is, "Don't throw away the garbage tonight and tell everyone to meet me by the trash bags at closing." At closing I would have every manager and aspiring manager assist me as I would go through the garbage. If you're a restaurant owner and you want to find out where all of your money is going, all you have to do is look in your trash cans. Whatever your patrons aren't eating is right there. It may look like bags of old food but what it really translates to is money. If your patrons didn't think it was worth eating then that means you either gave them too much or gave them something they did not want.

From the onset of the Atkin's Diet restaurants were losing money like crazy. When we would look through their trash we would find tons of bread, baked potatoes, french-fries, corn and spaghetti. The restaurant patrons weren't eating it and most restaurant owners would never have see it unless they looked in the trash; a task considered being beneath everyone except the busboys.

Back in the 1970's and early 1980's the slang term "bread" was used for money. You remember "lay some bread on me." Well all the restaurants that were shutting down left and right in 2002 and 2003 after the Atkin's Diet became popular must have forgotten ghetto analogy; otherwise, they would still be in business today.

Why did the meat and dairy industry sue Oprah Winfrey when she allowed a guest to appear on her show and say negative things about beef? Because one hour after the show aired, the meat and dairy people felt their pockets get a little lighter. The only way to make the food industry change is to hit them where it hurts - in their pockets. Don't get me wrong, if you are a business owner, I'm not attempting to shut you down. Adopting a healthy menu offers many advantages for you. Healthy customers live longer and use your services longer. Healthy employees work better and are happier. If you are a business owner stop allowing vendors to bring unhealthy products to your work site; such as sodas, candy bars, and transfat filled potato chips.

If you are an employee, stop buying the bad stuff and leave little notes on the vending machine with suggestions as to what you really would like such as granola bars and fresh fruit juices. The chain reaction here might amaze you. Watch and see your health care costs will go down while less people will call in sick for work, all of which will lessen the stress on both employee and employer.

A few years ago I ran into one of the Vice Presidents of the Kroger grocery store chain in a parking lot. She asked me to become a store manager for their company. It was attractive to me because I wanted to get away from traveling so much, to stay closer to my family and not have the burden of owning the entire store. I took the offer. During that time I became a store manager at the largest Kroger in the world which is located in one of the wealthiest areas in the world - Alpharetta, Georgia. The store is more than 80,000 square feet and at that time had more than 200 employees. The customer database list read like the Beverly Hills and Silicon Valley of the South. The parking lot was always filled with very expensive cars and the ladies who shopped there whore some of the largest diamond rings you ever saw. When a customer would come into the store to ask for something that we didn't have we would do everything in our power to get it.

One of the major reasons Kroger hired me was because of the increase in the demand of health food items. My background in the health industry made me a perfect fit, because this Kroger was their largest store it, also housed the company's largest health food department. The health food section was larger than most stand alone health food stores. Customer demand had caused the company to begin bringing in more and more health food items.

If we go to the grocery stores in our communities and begin nagging and hounding the managers with letters asking for organic items; they will be forced to comply with our demands. If you give this book to everyone you know; we can ignite a revolution.

Food groups get a taste of tea

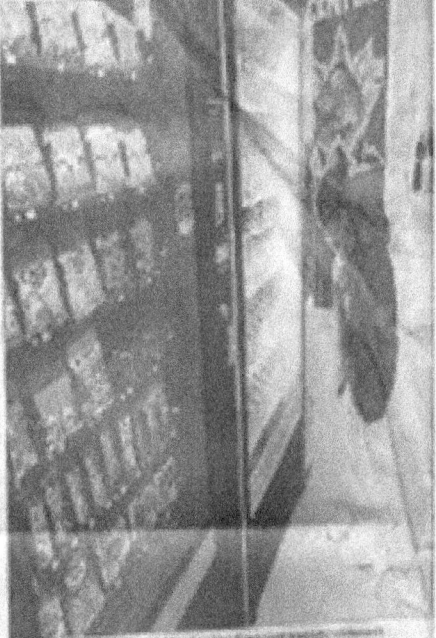

Why Organic? Why Supplements?

I want you to understand that organic food is the best food for you, if it is a clean food as recognized in the Bible. However, because of the lack of good soil as a whole, organic foods alone are not good enough. You still need to supplement your diet with vitamins and minerals from organic sources that come from companies that measure the quality of the contents of their products. By this I mean chemical tests that determine if the plants used in their ingredients are what the bottle says it is. These tests should show that no other substances have been placed in as fillers, and that the vitamin and mineral contents are what are stated.

You also want to be sure that the product is a water soluble plant source that will digest in your body.

Any supplement you get, you should place the first tablet or capsule into a glass of water to see if it will dissolve promptly or within two to four hours. You may stirs lightly every hour. The faster it dissolves or breaks into tiny pieces the faster it will work for you.

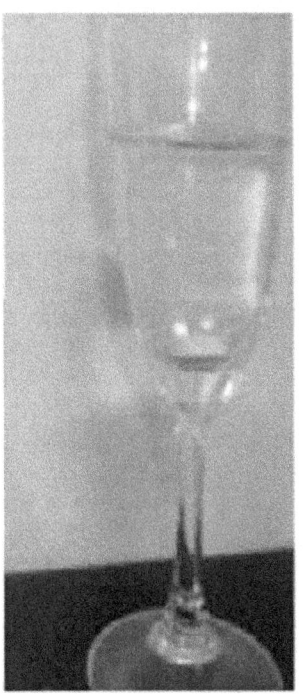 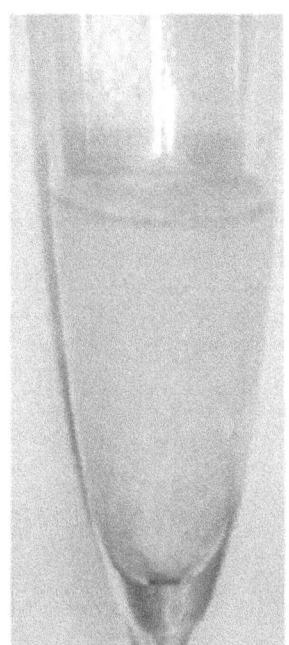

Let us talk about what you need on a daily basis. First and foremost because

calcium deficiencies cause the majority of the health problems we are plagued with

in the US and Europe, you should take the equivalent of 1500 mg a day. Half of

this each day should be in the form of live foods (such as greens, spinach or kale.)

The other half should be in the form of a plant source supplement. Next, you need

200 mcg of chromium and 25 mcg of vanadium which are both rare and important trace minerals that help your body process sugar. In as many as 99% of all the instances I have experienced these two minerals have made type 2 diabetes disappear within two months. The total absence of these two minerals in our diets is making diabetes one of the fastest growing diseases in our society. Only twenty years ago this disease was called "adult onset diabetes." Now we can't call it by that name anymore because it is now attacking children in their early teens on a widespread basis. In many cases some children are showing signs of it in their preteen years.

If you are a Christian, you may ask - "Why should I begin my study on how I should eat in the Old Testament?" The answer is for the same reason the early church searched the Holy Scriptures daily. (Acts 17:11) They were searching the only Scriptures available at the time, the Old Testament. They were putting to test the teachings of the Apostle Paul, to see if his words measured up to what was taught in these Scriptures. The New Testament was built upon the Old Testament.

When the Apostle Paul wrote his second letter to a young evangelist named Timothy, he told him to *"continue in the things you have learned and become convinced of, knowing from whom you have learned them; and that from childhood you have known the Sacred Writings (Old Testament) which are able to give you the wisdom that leads to salvation through faith which is in Christ Jesus."* (2 Timothy 3:24-25) Now notice Verses 16-17 - *"ALL SCRIPTURE (New Testament was not complied yet) is INSPIRED BY GOD and profitable for teaching, for reproof, for correction, for training in righteousness; that the man of God may be adequate, equipped for every good work."*

In the book of Daniel we find the belief that unclean foods can defile a person.

Notice Daniel 1:8 - *"But Daniel made up his mind that he would not defile himself with the king's choice of food or with the wine which he drank; so he sought permission from the commander of the officials that he might not defile himself."*

Daniel clearly believed King Nebuchadnezzar's choice of food would be bad for him. Daniel was a prophet. He had the indwelling of the Holy Spirit of God in him. He believed the Gentile's food would harm his body. Daniel gave his request to be spared the King's meat, and to be served only vegetables and water for ten days. Shadrach, Meshach and Abednego also requested the same. Their outward appearance was to be checked at the end of the ten days to see if they looked healthy.

Notice Verse 15 -*"And at the end often days their APPEARANCE seemed better and they were fatter than all the youths who had been eating the king's choice food."*

Cleanse First

Have you ever heard the saying "what goes up must come down?" Well in the same way, what goes in must come out. Most people do not like talking about this subject but herein lays the key to optimal health. This may get a little graphic so prepare your stomachs and your minds.

Do you have one or two bowel movements a week? What about once or twice a day? Well the majority of us feel that bowel elimination once a day is okay. Some of you feel that two or three times a week is okay for you because your system is "different." Well, the truth of the matter is that you should have bowel elimination for every meal that you consume. This includes a meal as small as a banana or an apple for breakfast. Think about it for a moment. Infants eat then eliminate. Then they eat again and eliminate. So I ask you- what's changed between infancy and adulthood? I'll tell you - our diets! Early in life our system digests only milk. Then when we are older, we introduced real food. Our system says: Okay, I can handle this. Then we introduce vegetables. This is great, cereal and vegetables. Next is fruit. Well the fruit is fine unless you combine them with cereal (carbs) or vegetables. Fruit should always be eaten alone or with other fruit. Babies are fine in the beginning but eventually they get gas. Then later the bowel movements are less frequent.

Let me explain: Fruit digests in about thirty minutes or less if eaten alone. When eaten with other foods like carbs, vegetables, or proteins, processing slows down. These other foods take longer to digest. When you eat the fruit with them, the fruit does not digest immediately. Instead fermentation begins, which causes gas and bloating. As we get older, our digestive system strengthens and we are able to process the food better but at a cost. It costs our body by causing large stomachs, hemorrhoids, gas, bloating, constipation, and even death. It also costs our skin by causing acne, eczema, psoriasis, and even cancer. Believe it or not, it costs our minds as well.

Are you sometimes angry or frustrated and not sure why? Have you noticed that, after a good bowel movement, your mood changes for the better? You are happy and feel a sense of relief. Most of you would probably agree that you would prefer not to be around someone experiencing constipation and road rage or constipation and post partum depression. You probably want to run for your life. And men, have you ever stopped to think (I know most of you don't) that maybe all those times you thought your wife or girlfriend was "PMS-ing", maybe she just needed to take a good relaxing (bowel movement).

Now all jokes aside, bowel elimination is one of the most important functions of the body. It affects your mind, body and spirit and the lack thereof can lead to death. "Many cancers and disease that lead to death begin in the colon. (VegetarianTimes 1998) Without proper elimination, our bodies are not able to absorb all the nutrients in the food we eat. Now as if it wasn't bad enough that our soil was already depleted, imagine not being able to absorb all the nutrients you do get from your foods and supplements. Do you know you could have fecal matter in your body from years ago? Taking an over the counter laxative will not do enough for you. The body needs fiber and a thorough cleansing program at least twice a year. You take the time to clean the outside but the inside is much more important. Remember, looks can be deceiving. You can look like a supermodel or star athlete on the outside but could house all kinds of disease and deficiencies in the inside.

Now that we know how important bowel elimination is to the body, let's talk about having"healthy" bowel elimination.

Good bowel elimination should not be runny, heavy like a sinker, or long and skinny like a pencil. It should be full, 6 to 12 inches long and it should float on top of the water. Guess what else? It should not stink. Can you believe that? Bowel that do not stink (Humm). When you exit the bathroom after having a good healthy movement, the next person to enter should not come out holding their nose or gagging.

Healthy bowel movements come from eating foods in their proper food order, and by eating plenty of the right foods, such as fresh fruits, and by drinking plenty of water providing your colon has been properly cleansed. If you haven't heard you should be drinking about sixteen 8 oz. glasses of filtered water a day. This allows your body to perform optimal cleaning each day.

Together the small and large intestines are over 20 feet long. Imagine having over 20 feet of fecal matter decaying along the walls of your intestines for decades. This decay prohibits the intestines from absorbing all the nutrients from the food you eat as well as from your supplements. Over time, this turns into disease and can lead to cancer. So don't feel inconvenienced when you need to have a bowel movement, even if you are at work. Take the time and feel blessed and relieved in knowing that your body is cleansing itself. Make sure you cleanse the inside of your body at least twice a year with one of the following super cleansers. Also, stay regular by eating right, drinking plenty of water and doing abdominal exercises.

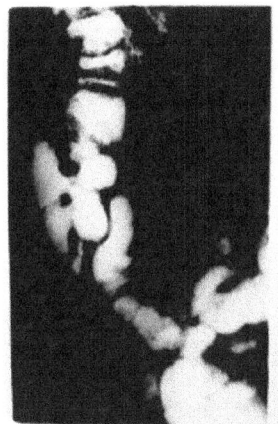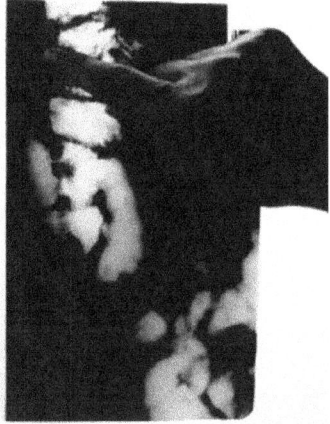

Over the years I have worked with many herbal based cleansing programs but the most effective one I've come across wad the Symmetry cleanse Bundle. It has two parts the BotanaCleanse and the ParaCleanse.

With BotanaCleanse your body will receive a gentle mild cleansing with botanicals and natural fibers. It will also provide the colon with probiotics to support the "friendly flora" in the body. It usually takes about 11 days to complete and it should be taken every three months to six months.   ParaCleanse is the second part of the Cleanse-Bundle. According to the CDC 85-95% of the population is living with parasites! It is possible to have these damaging organisms and not even know it; however you may know or have the symptoms, digestive problems, allergy symptoms, impaired vision, menstrual irregularities, numbness in the hands, anemia, and general lethargy. These are just some of the damaging effects your body suffers from living with parasite contamination. The best way I've found to rid your body of possible parasites is with ParaCleanse. Its two phase system works to eliminate impurities in the first phase and nourishes the blood in the second phase. It also serves as a support system for your body's natural immune function.

So remember, thoroughly cleanse four times a year and make sure you have regular bowel movements, three a day, for a fitter, happier, healthier you.

Conclusion

It's time for a change. Make your voices heard and your choices known. Demand healthier snacks in the workplace, ask your grocer for more organic choices. We can make a difference. We wanted healthier fast food and now "Burger King" carries a Veggie Burger, McDonald's sells Asian salads with beans and fruit, Wendy's carries subs and Chick-fil-A offers free range chicken free of hormones and now they offer fruit cups, too.

If you are a person blessed to not have any serious illness or disease, you are probably saying, "I'm fine. I really don't need any supplements or anything." Maybe you have mild allergies, low energy, occasional forgetfulness, slight obesity, or a little digestive problem here and there. Maybe you have a low desire for romance or poor performance in the bedroom. These are key signs. Everyone needs supplements.

If it has been raining on your head, it's time to prevent this from turning into a tidal wave. You should start by taking "Genesis." It is a delicious combination of highly standardized fruit juices and whole fruit extracts, infused with a proprietary blend of herbs and other powerful foods. The renowned antioxidant properties of whole fruit pomegranate and whole fruit red grape combine with the healing and restorative nature of whole fruit apple, olive leaf and Aloe Vera for a heavenly-tasting 100% juice product.

Symmetry has chosen to use the slow but powerful infusion process with Genesis to create the greatest concentration of protective anthropalexins (literally, "protector of humankind"), age-fighting antioxidants and powerful phytonutrients imaginable.

Infusion is the lost art and science of coaxing maximum benefits from botanical materials without adding damaging heat or nasty chemicals. Infusion has been practiced for thousands of years and has been the basis for nearly all medications.

Do you know what the #1 cause of death is in America? It's heart disease. Heart disease strikes and kills almost every 45 seconds; many victims have no history or signs of heart problems. Don't let this be you. Ever heard the saying "An apple a day will help keep the doctor away."? Well today, it takes more than just an apple which today is probably filled with pesticides, wax, and artificial coloring and grown from depleted soil. What you need now is an organic apple a day times two and one of two supplement called Mega Chel and CardioEssentials.

Mega Chel and CardoEssentials contain natural supplements that have a powerhouse of nutrients to support the entire circulatory system. The B vitamins and panothenic acid for the nervous system, CoQ 10, gingko biloba, and Hawthorne for the heart and circulation as well as a host of others like: Iron, magnesium, and potassium just to name a few. One of my customers had experienced four heart attacks over the past three years. We put him on Mega Chel. A week later he had his fifth heart attack. The doctors had warned him that the next one may kill him because of all the damage that had taken place in his heart. The doctors were amazed to find out that his heart had actually started to mend itself. Since that trip to the hospital five years ago, he hasn't been back to the hospital and all he has been taking is his daily two doses of Mega-Chel.

In today's society, we are bombarded with fast foods, high stress, and high tech stuff everywhere. We don't take the time to cook healthy, breathe healthy air, or exercise. This combination will kill you and is killing us by storming numbers. It is raining on your health. The Rainmen are coming! Shelter yourself from the rain. Take the things that I'm telling you about and go to our website http://www.rainbowdiet.org/. There you'll find a list of all the latest health information I have to offer and what I advise everyone to take on a daily basis. The products listed are ones either I or my clients have tried with great results. Also everything listed comes from companies that actually test their products for purity and pesticide residue. You don't have to buy these products from me but I ask that you douse these products. They will protect your family the way they have protected mine. If you do choose to buy them through our web site I would like to thank you in advance your patronage will allows us to continue doing what we do - that is helping you and others maintain good health.

Remember this book and spread the word. Don't keep the knowledge in your head. Use it to keep yourself ahead and healthy in life. Protect yourself from the storm of the Rainmen (Doctors,FDA, Grocers, and Pharmacists) with an umbrella policy of "Protection 4 Life" Protection 4 Life with Ultra Vitality & Genesis is a great beginning for a healthful, energetic lifestyle! Vitamins, minerals, antioxidants, and other necessary nutrients will keep your body functioning at its optimum. You can get it at: www.rainbowdiet.org

I'll end this with a joke that I once heard a comedian tell on Comedy Central. There is a lot of truth to it. "In Life you only have two things you really have to worry about; so get all the other things out of your mind and relax. Every morning when you wake up all you have to worry about is two things whether you are healthy or sick. If you are healthy, then you're fine and you can go on with your business. If you are sick, then you only have two things to worry about, that's, are you going to get better or worse? If you get better than you have nothing else to worry about. If you get worse you have two things to worry about - whether you are going to get better or die. If you get better, then you've got nothing else to worry about, but if you die, you've got two things to worry about – that's Heaven or Hell. If you go to Heaven, you've got nothing else to worry about, but if you go to Hell, you've got two things to worry about- that's original or extra crispy.

Now here is the more serious note. When it's all said and done, what's it all worth to you? If you live a few years longer, if you don't do anything with it? I learned a long time ago that the reason we are put here on earth to embark upon this journey called life is to help others - our family members, our loved ones and those people we pass every day on our journey. Use this time to find Christ if you haven't already and if you have found Him, help someone else find Him. Show the eating habits he practiced so they can experience Him to the fullest. You've seen the bracelets that say, "W.W.J.D," "What Would Jesus Do." Well, what would Jesus Eat.

Don't use the contents of this book to chastise someone, but calmly tell them of your experiences. Don't offend your brother: *Proverbs 18:19 A brother offended is harder to be won than a strong city: and their contentions are like the bars of a castle.*

Questions and Other Materials

Inevitably you will encounter people who will try to discredit it the things you have read in this book. So, I've taken the liberty to go over a few probable situations. There are a few other sections in the Bible which ministers will attempt to throw at you.

In Acts 10 Peter was given a dream about unclean animals and was told to kill and eat (verse13)   *11 He saw heaven opened and something like a large sheet being let down to earth by its four corners. 12 It contained all kinds of four-footed animals, as well as reptiles of the earth and birds of the air. 13 Then a voice told him, "Get up, Peter. Kill and eat."*

He refused, because he had never eaten any-thing common or unclean, but he is commanded two more times. Later the meaning is revealed:

15 "Do not call anything impure that God has made clean."

When three non-Jews show up at his door that had given their lives to Christ and wanted to hear more about Jesus. Peter knew that he must let them into his home, something that he would not have done before because they were unclean.

28 "God has shown me that I should not call any man impure or unclean."

The food could not make his heart or love for Christ unclean. The vision was telling Peter that clean and unclean didn't matter when it came to your soul. Both were now welcome in Christ.

About the Authors

Carl Millender is a health and business consultant in the City of Atlanta. His business clients include Wal*Mart and Coke. As a health consultant, he has been a consultant to many celebrities - such as Keith L. Brown. In his spare time he likes to produce visual media. Since 2002 he has produced and directed three feature movies Family Curse, Rejectors of the Blood of Christ, Positive, For Honor or Glory, The Good Ole Days, SB1070, Secret Societies of Slavery and At Mamu's Feet.

His natural path training has been as an apprentice under Dr. Janet Adams-Urquhart and Dr. Wiletha Williams. He has been helping people find a better, more healthy way to live since 1994. He and Shelia have appeared on talk shows on both television and radio since that time and have helped thousands of people.

In April 1999, they created the herbal supplement, Metabocharge, which has helped to give people the extra energy they need on a daily basis as an alternative to coffee and soda.

In March 2005 Carl and Shelia launched the Enjoy Life program where for only $850, a nutritionist will guide a client through an entire day of healthy living in their own home. The client learns how to shop for healthy food and create daily meals and snacks in accordance to God's laws. Call (678)698-1970 for questions about the program.

The Millender family has a rich history in America. Carl's great uncle Robert Millender was a famous Civil Rights lawyer in the city of Detroit Michigan where the Millender Center is named after him. In the Mid 1900's his other great uncle Lucky Millender was blazing the International Jazz scene with the Lucky Millender Orchestra. The Millender family is also featured in The Smithsonian Institute as the first American family of African descent to start a formal business in the United States.

Gloria Millender, Carl's mother is an author in her own regard, but is most known as an educator in the state of Louisiana and has won numerous awards for her excellence.

Order Today

The Protection for life with Genesis and Ultra Vitality Kit

- The Cookbook

- Live DVD

- 2 Audio CD's

- 1 Mega Chel

- 1 Noni

- 1 SugarReg

- 1 Liquid Calcium

- 1 Colloidal Minerals

- a bonus copy.

$249.99 Order

The Enjoy Life Health Assistant Program - Need help getting started with your healthy new life then call us. For only $850 we'll have a personal consultant guide you around for an entire 16 hour day. They will help you shop, cook, and prepare healthy snacks for you or your family. Just call Shelia at (678) 508-3549 to setup a program date.

Recommended Reading

ANGER IN THE NORTH - This book is truly God's warning to the church —the end is coming and it is surely the time to take heed to God's message! This book will inform, educate, and stimulate your spirituality! It's great! Linda Andrews is trying to raise her 10-year-old gifted musician son on a waitress salary. This may not seem to be unusual until a mystery unfolds when we find out that Linda has an amazing gift of her own. A wonderful gift held prisoner within her due to the shadows of her past that torment her. A past she feels responsible for. Along comes our hero, Julian Noel, to help Linda break free from this prison- a prison of fear and guilt. But will he be too late as the shadows of her past begin to take form and hunt Linda down... Sometimes you may believe that the final pages to your life's story have already been written. Sometimes you may believe that your actions have been the ink that penned the pages. Sometimes you may believe that nothing in those pages can be altered. But because of the Greater Love - The perceived end is not the end.

ANGER
IN THE NORTH

*A Warning
for the Church*

Gloria B. Millender

Preface by John G. Griffin

Bibliography

Elias Marilyn. Suicide Alert Has Parents Rethinking Anti-Depressants USA Today 2005 Feb 11 DMcCoy, Kevin. Drug Maker Rebuffed Called to Monitor Users. USA Today 2004, December 71D

Jensen, Bernard, D.C. Tissue Cleansing Through Bowel Management Escondido, CA 92029: Hidden Valley, 1981 Starfield, Dr. Barbara, M.D. MPH.

 Is US Health Really the Best in the World, JAMA 2000; July 26- 284, 483-485EPA Team Report. Genes from Biotech grass Scatter for Miles USA Today 2004 September 23 1 D

Bible Gateway.com New King James Version (Genesis 2:16,17-3:1-8,15-19) (1 Corinthians 3:16,14:33) (Leviticus 25:1-8, 17:1) (Exodus 34:26) (1Timothy 6:10) (2 Timothy 3:24-25) (Ecclesiastes10:19) (Daniel 1:8-10)

US Senate Bill #264 . Land Mineral Salts Depletion. Cosmopolitan Magazine 1936

Pope John Paul II lent 1993 Speech

Schurmann, Franz "Sands of Time: Earth's Expanding Deserts Can't Be Stopped," The Pacific News Service, Commentary, San Francisco, CA 2005, Apr06

Brown, Lester. Shrinking Farmland China The Globalist Magazine 2004, March 12

Josephson, Elmer. God's Key to Health and Happiness

O.T. Diet Regulations and Health Epstein, Gady A. "China dinner delicacies succumb to SARS." Guangzhou, China.

Baltimore Sun 2003 May 14

CFIA. The Animal and Plant Health Risk Assessment Network, and the Canadian Food Inspection Agency, located in Nepean, Ontario, Canada 2003-2004

Leaf, Alexander M.D. Everyday is a Blessing When You're Over a 100 New York, National Geograph-ics1973

January Sherman, Paul PhD., Lactose Intolerance Linked To Ancestral Environment, Cornell University, Ithaca, NY 2005 June 2 Neergaad Lauran.

Millions at Risk From Osteoporosis Washington D.C., Star Tribune 2004 Oct 15

Hellmich, Nancy. "The French Diet Connection" Paris, France USA Today 2005, January 4

Schweitzer, Albert PhD, M.D. Philosophy of Civilization Gabon, Africa 1923 C. T.

Campion [Buffalo: Prometheus, 1987], 307-29Price, Dr. Weston M.D. PhD. DDS.

Nutrition and Physical Degeneration Radiant Life, 1923

Campbell, Dr. T. Colin PhD. "The China Study." China-Oxford-Cornell Health

Project Benbella Books 2005 Herlin, Dr. Susan J. 2003 Ancient African

Civilizations to ca. 1500: Pharaonic Egypt to Ca. 800 BC, p 27.

Correct Food Order Meals

When trying meal suggestions, we encourage you to use organic ingredients when possible and use a veggie or soy substitute for any dairy product when at all possible.

For your health and enjoyment, we have included some helpful meal suggestions. Remember to eat fruit by itself and wait thirty minutes before eating anything else. When eating your meals, we also encourage you to properly combine your foods; eating meat with vegetables and starches with vegetables. Do not combine meat and starches for best digestion and quicker absorption. We have also included some of our favorite recipes. We hope you enjoy!

Meal Suggestions

Breakfast Suggestions

Smoothies

Raw fruit

Cereal with Rice or Almond Milk

Omelet w/veggies and veggie cheese

Herbal tea and a slice of toast

Soy yogurt

Orange Juice followed by turkey bacon and turkey sausage

Granola Yeast free waffles Grits (Soy margarine)

Red potatoes and onions

Multigrain pancakes Tofu scramble

Lunch and Dinner Suggestions

Tuna Salad on Romaine Lettuce

Stir fry Chicken and Vegetables

Grilled Salmon and Salad

Spaghetti with sauce and veggie Parmesan cheese (No meat)

Veggie Lasagna with corn on the cob

Salmon patties w/ broccoli

Veggie fried rice w/spring or egg roll

Lentil soup w/ Spinach salad

Lemon Pepper wingettes w/favorite veggie (broccoli, carrots, asparagus)

Turkey cutlets w/gravy (cook like "Pork chops") green bean casserole, squash

Lettuce Wraps w/ Chicken

Veggie Pita with Tuna Salad, Chicken Salad

Chicken Wrap (With veggie tortilla)

Mongolian Beef (Soy protein) w/onions and veggie curry pockets

Blackbean Soup with Salad

Curry chicken with sautéed asparagus

Barbecue chicken, deviled eggs and a small salad

Mashed potatoes with Spinach and glazed carrots

Chili made with ground turkey and side salad

Omelet w/veggies and veggie cheese

Barbecue (soy) beef ribs grilled corn on the cob and baked beans

Bistro beef (soy protein) and sautéed mushrooms

Snack suggestions

Fruit Salad (Eaten Alone)

Raw veggies and dip Protein bar

Nuts (Cashew, peanuts, pistachios, etc.)

Popcorn

Soy yogurt

Veggie chips (they are delicious)

Sorbet (Not sherbet)

Raisins

Natural fruit leather strips

Millender Favorites

Rainbow Smoothie

1 banana

1/2 cup of strawberries

1/2 cup of pineapples,

1 mango,

1 cup of apple juice

Blend all the ingredients together in a blender for 2 minutes and serve.

<u>Rainbow Omelet</u>

2 eggs,

1 tablespoon onions

1 tablespoon green peppers

2 tablespoon of soy margarine

1/2 cup of salsa or veggie cheese

Salt

Pepper

Beat 2 eggs in a bowl and salt and pepper to taste. Put soy margarine in small frying pan on medium heat. Sprinkle the onions and green pepper evenly. When egg is cooked on one side, add cheese if desired and fold egg in half. Let sit for 30 seconds and then turn to other side. Let cook another 30 seconds and serve. For those of you that love southwestern flavor, pour salsa over the omelet and enjoy!!

Lemon Pepper Chicken

1 pack of chicken wingettes

Lemon pepper seasoning

2 tablespoon soy margarine

Salt

Pepper

1/2 lemon

Seasoned wingettes with salt and pepper to taste. Place in Non-stick pan and cover. Then, place wingettes into oven preheated at 350 degrees. Let cook for 30 minutes then sprinkle with lemon pepper seasoning and turn over each piece and sprinkle the other side. Let bake for another 30 minutes. Now pour the melted soy margarine over the wingettes and cook uncovered for 15 minutes. Squeeze fresh lemon over wingettes and enjoy. Serve with Celery Sticks, raw veggies and dip or steamed broccoli (our favorite)

Veggie Lasagna

1 package of Lasagna, uncooked

26oz Organic Pasta Sauce

3 tablespoon olive oil

2 tablespoon soy margarine

3 medium squash

1 medium onion

12oz package of spinach frozen

1/4 cup fresh parsley

1 cup of shredded mozzarella cheese (veggie)

1/2 cup parmesan cheese (veggie)

16oz firm tofu

1 5oz ricotta cheese

Salt

Pepper

1) Cook pasta according to directions on the box.

2) Cook spinach in 2 tbsp of soy margarine and a pinch of salt and pepper. Set aside.

3) Sauté squash and onions in olive oil until ten-der. Add pasta sauce, parsley and stir. In another bowl mix the ricotta cheese, 1 cup mozzarella and the parmesan cheese together. Heat oven to 350 degrees.

4) Spread 1/3 of sauce on bottom of 1 3x9x2 inch baking dish. Place 3 pieces of pasta over the sauce mixture. Spread 1/2 of cheese mixture over pasta. Cover cheese mixture with 1/2 of the spin-ach.

5) If you like tofu, this is a great time to add it to the lasagna. Cut tofu into small chunks, season, cook by boiling and place into the lasagna. Re-peat step 4 then top with remaining pasta pieces and cover with remaining sauce; sprinkle with left over mozzarella and parmesan cheese. Cover with foil and bake 45 minutes. Let it stand15 minutes before serving. This recipe is great with a side salad. Enjoy!!